# AFTA SpringerBriefs in Family Therapy



**Series Editor**

Carmen Knudson-Martin
Education & Counseling, Rogers Hall
Lewis & Clark Grad School
Portland, OR, USA

SpringerBriefs present concise summaries of cutting-edge research and practical applications. Featuring compact volumes of 50 to 125 pages, the series covers a range of content from professional to academic. Typical topics might include: A timely report of state-of-the art analytical techniques A bridge between new research results, as published in journal articles, and a contextual literature review A snapshot of a hot or emerging topic An in-depth case study or clinical example A presentation of core concepts that students must understand in order to make independent contributions

More information about this series at http://www.springer.com/series/11846

marcela polanco • Navid Zamani
Christina Da Hee Kim
Editors

# Bilingualism, Culture, and Social Justice in Family Therapy

Springer

AFTA
American Family Therapy Academy

*Editors*
marcela polanco
College of Education
San Diego State University
San Diego, CA, USA

Navid Zamani
College of Education
San Diego State University
San Diego, CA, USA

Christina Da Hee Kim
License to Freedom
El Cajon, CA, USA

ISSN 2196-5528 ISSN 2196-5536 (electronic)
AFTA SpringerBriefs in Family Therapy
ISBN 978-3-030-66035-2 ISBN 978-3-030-66036-9 (eBook)
https://doi.org/10.1007/978-3-030-66036-9



This Springer imprint is published by the registered company Springer Nature Switzerland AG
The registered company address is: Gewerbestrasse 11, 6330 Cham, Switzerland

# Series Editor Foreword

The AFTA Springer Briefs in Family Therapy is an official publication of the American Family Therapy Academy. Each volume focuses on the practice and policy implications of innovative systemic research and theory in family therapy and allied fields. Our goal is to make information about families and systemic practices in societal contexts widely accessible in a reader friendly, conversational, and practical style. AFTA's core commitment to equality, social responsibility, and justice are represented in each volume.

In *Bilingualism, Culture, and Social Justice in Family Therapy,* editors marcela polanco, Navid Zamani, and Christina Da Hee Kim have pulled together the wisdom and creativity of 25 authors who each practice family therapy across the boundaries of language. Their accounts voice their experiences and expertise moving from one language to another "in split seconds" in the service of their clients. Because family therapy, like other mental health professions, is produced and taught within a monolingual paradigm that centers Anglo concepts and English, the authors make visible what has not been recognized and articulated within the field—that bilingual practice is not "simply" an act of translation, but instead involves traversing culturally specific identities and meanings embedded in language that are not translatable.

As a monolingual family therapy educator and researcher, reading this volume opened a previously unexplored world through which the linguistic concepts and practices I teach and study perpetuate discrimination and racism, and have a colonizing effect. Bilingual practitioners have been left on their own to draw on their intuition, intention, capacity to improvise, and their communities to negotiate ethical, equitable professional practice. *Bilingualism, Culture, and Social Justice in Family Therapy* is a step toward awareness and accountability within the field that, as the editors state, will promote movement "whereby the current standard English training curriculums, therapy frameworks, journals, and professional conferences would shift to resemble the multiple languages represented" in our communities. Bilingual and monolingual readers alike will be inspired with a call for reflection and transformative action.

AFTA Springer Briefs in Family Therapy Carmen Knudson-Martin
Lewis & Clark College,
Portland, OR, USA

# Foreword

We are very pleased to have been invited to write this preface because this book, in some ways, is a continuation of the conversation we had in the early 1990s about bilingual therapists' challenges of navigating the multiple linguistic and cultural voices in family therapy consultations. Our conversations resulted in the development of the nationally recognized Psychological Services for Spanish Speaking Populations (PSSSP) training that has trained hundreds of family therapists and psychologists over the last two decades. We are proud that one of the editors of the book in hand, marcela polanco, was the Director of the PSSSP program for a time in the mid-2010s. The PSSSP program is also represented here by its current director Carlos Ramos, a former faculty member, Jimena Castro, and a graduate of the PSSSP program, Joseph Guerrero.

*I really enjoyed your class, though when I was home* [in México] *over Christmas break, I didn't have the language to explain what I learned to my friends who are mothers.*

This reflection was from a student from Mexico City after my (JLB) first semester of teaching at Our Lady of the Lake University (OLLU). As monolingual English speakers, we were puzzled by this statement. We had no way of understanding why someone who was a native Spanish speaker was unable to translate what she had learned in English to Spanish. In subsequent conversations with colleagues and Spanish speaking students, we became aware of the complexity of applying learnings in one language to working in a second language; that language in which learning occurs may limit its application in another language. Inevitably, theories and ideas that professionals master in one language are often not accessible in conversations in another language, regardless of the speaker's proficiency in each language. The direct translation of ideas and concepts creates other challenges. They are necessarily linguistically and culturally unique and meanings are rarely equivalent in both languages. Further, constructs derived from theoretical approaches originating in English may be difficult to use when working in other languages and cultures. For example, the meaning of "the self" is not easily translated into Spanish as the construct of "the self," as we use it in English does not exist in many Latinx cultures.

Applying what they learned in English to working with clients in Spanish was an even bigger challenge for our students who were heritage speakers of Spanish. This dilemma was described by Aguirre (2004):

> I feel inadequate because I sometimes do not have all of the right words and expressions readily available when I do therapy in Spanish. You see, although I am bilingual, I know that my capabilities in Spanish vocabulary are very much lacking. I learned the therapeutic language in English, but I do not readily have those same words and phrases in Spanish (pp. 9–10).

We learned that mere conversational proficiency in a language was not sufficient for competent mental health practice in that language. Professionals who intended to practice in a language other than the language they were trained in needed training to bridge the gap between conversational fluency and professional proficiency. These discussions eventually led us to develop OLLU's pioneering PSSSP specialization in the graduate psychology and marriage and family therapy programs (Biever et al. 2011). The PSSSP program's goal is to graduate students who are equally competent to provide psychological services in both Spanish and English. The PSSSP program supports students in the development of professional proficiency in Spanish in various ways. Biever and Santos (2016) interviewed graduates of the PSSSP program about how the program had affected their professional development. One graduate reported that the PSSSP faculty assisted them to "push past the fear of saying something wrong or being embarrassed…knowing that the people that would help me with the training, the people that I was working with, weren't going to make fun of me." Another noted "I was a hesitant to get in the PSSSP because I thought my Spanish was very rusty, and then I got in the program and I think it helped me feel more comfortable speaking Spanish and also feel competent being able to do therapy in Spanish." PSSSP graduates described how the experience of training on Spanish-speaking teams[1] with live supervision facilitated their learning about using clients' language and idioms and increased their Spanish therapeutic vocabulary. These teams provided the supportive context and opportunities to increase their confidence in conducting therapy in Spanish and practicing Spanish. The PSSSP program helps students who are heritage speakers of Spanish develop proficiency in both speaking and writing in Spanish. For example, one student noted: "Spanish is my first language but it was my social language, so academically I wasn't the best writer in Spanish, but she [Spanish instructor] helped me develop all of my writing skills in Spanish, as well." Another student described how the PSSSP contributed to her confidence in conducting therapy in Spanish:

> When I do therapy in Spanish, I use the proper concepts and terms and know that there is a difference as I'm trying to deliver my intervention. When I've been around other people who don't have the training, I know that they're very competent in English, but it does not translate in Spanish.

[1] For a detailed description of how we use a team approach to training graduate students, please see Bobele et al (2008).

This book is a welcome addition to the ongoing conversation about how language shapes the delivery and transformation of family therapy in the USA. The editors' intention to "document stories about the intricacies of the languages bilingual family therapists speak in their lives and practices" has been met and exceeded in our opinion.

These stories of individual therapists from diverse cultural backgrounds dealing with adapting English originating practices to their preferred language and culture opens new windows into creative practices. This book will be an intriguing starting point for family therapists struggling with the paradoxes of learning their craft in English and the challenge of applying that learning in their originating language. The chapter authors set the stage for work that addresses the wider question of "What is the relationship between the originating language of the theories of family therapy and the languages of the culture that adopt these theories?". For example, family therapy is taught in Spain where textbooks, readings, supervision, and clients are all fluent in Spanish. However, many of the originating theories in family therapy are Eurocentric without respect to the languages that disseminate these theories. We are hoping the current collection of essays opens a broader discussion about the dominance of Eurocentric thinking on our helping practices with non-European cultures.

Our Lady of the Lake University Monte Bobele
San Antonio, TX, USA
Our Lady of the Lake University Joan Biever
San Antonio, TX, USA

## References

Aguirre, C. (2004). One Latina's path through marriage and family therapy training. *Journal of Feminist Family Therapy, 16*(1), 1–17.

Biever, J. L., Gómez, J. P., González, C. G., & Patrizio, M. (2011). Psychological services to Spanish-Speaking populations: A model curriculum for training competent professionals. *Training and Education in Professional Psychology, 5*, 81–87. https://doi.org/10.1037/a0023535.

Biever, J. L., & Santos, J. (2016). Ofreciendo terapia en el idioma de preferencia del cliente: El modelo de preparacion profesional calificada en dos idiomas de OLLU (Providing therapy in the client's preferred language: the OLLU model for professional competence in two language). In L. Charlés & G. Samarasinghe, *Family therapy in global humanitarian contexts* (pp 51–63). New York, NY: Springer.

Bobele, M., Lopez, S. S.-G., Scamardo, M., & Solórzano, B. (2008). Single-session/walk-in therapy with Mexican-American clients. *Journal of Systemic Therapies, 27*, 75–89.

# Contents

# Contributors

**Gricelda Alvarez** San Diego, CA, USA

**Jimena Castro** Department of Psychology, Our Lady of the Lake University, San Antonio, TX, USA

**Mu-Lan Chau** Associate Marriage and Family Therapist, Riverside, CA, USA

**Wonyoung L. Cho** Marriage, Couples, and Family Therapy, Lewis & Clark Graduate School of Education and Counseling, Portland, OR, USA

Lewis & Clark College, Portland, OR, USA

**Diana K. Chung** Community Health and Private Practice, Alhambra, CA, USA

**Mohammed Darbi** License to Freedom, El Cajon, CA, USA

**Letti Estrella** SDSU Center for Community Counseling and Engagement CCCE, SDSU Centro de Consejería para la Comunidad CCCE, San Diego, CA, USA

**Joseph Alvaro Guerrero Velez** Nova Southeastern University, Fort Lauderdale, FL, USA

**Ingrid Guerrieri** Christie's Place, San Diego, CA, USA

**Lodovica Guidarelli** Narrative Initiatives San Diego, San Diego, CA, USA

**Lorraine Hogan** Marriage and Family Therapist, San Diego, CA, USA

**Nidya Ramirez Ibarra** San Diego, CA, USA

**Christina Da Hee Kim** License to Freedom, El Cajon, CA, USA

**Jenny Leverman** License to Freedom, El Cajon, CA, USA

**Blanca Lizbeth Lugo** Private Practice, San Diego State University, San Diego, CA, USA

**Candea Mosley** License to Freedom, El Cajon, CA, USA

**Elvia Murga** San Diego, CA, USA

**Rocio Ocampo-Giancola** Private Practice, San Diego, CA, USA

**Daniel O'Sullivan** Narrative Initiatives of San Diego, San Diego, CA, USA

**Thien T. Pham** Private Practice, San Francisco, CA, USA

**marcela polanco** Marriage and Family Therapy Master's Program & Spanglish/Ingleñol Family Therapy Certificado, San Diego State University, San Diego, CA, USA

**Carlos A. Ramos** Our Lady of the Lake University, San Antonio, TX, USA

**Meg Rogers** License to Freedom, El Cajon, CA, USA

**Tisha X** Associate Marriage and Family Therapist, Riverside, CA, USA

**Eureka Vaughn** ChildNet Youth & Family Services, Long Beach, CA, USA

**Nadia Zamani** Marriage and Family Therapy, San Diego, CA, USA

**Navid Zamani** San Diego State University, San Diego, CA, USA

# About the Editors

**marcela polanco** is a Colombian immigrant in the United States. Her ancestry is African, Muisca, and South-European Colombian. She speaks Colombian Spanish, Immigrant English and Spanglish. As a family therapist, she is part of the faculty team of the Master's in Marriage and Family Therapy and the Spanglish/*Ingleñol* Family Therapy *Certificado* at San Diego State University located in unceded Kumeyaay land.

**Navid Zamani** is a Persian-American (Farsi and English-speaking) licensed marriage and family therapist practicing in San Diego. His work is structured around supporting families experiencing domestic violence, and conceptualizes these experiences from a post-structural, decolonial feminism situated in narrative practices. His interests in counseling, philosophy, and music are blended together with an interest in relational ethics, the politics of revolutionary love, and leaning into complexity. He currently teaches at San Diego State University and is the head of clinical services at License to Freedom, a non-profit organization that supports refugees and immigrants from the Middle East who are experiencing domestic violence issues.

**Christina Da Hee Kim** is a Korean immigrant who grew up in Los Angeles. She traverses between the worlds of English, Korean, and the mix of two languages, Konglish. Her interest in all forms of communication, including various languages and the non-verbal communication, stems from her exposure to Spanish-, Japanese-, and sign language-speaking worlds. As a recent graduate from the marriage and family therapy program at San Diego State University, she hopes to collaborate and explore relational ethics in diverse relationship dynamics from a postmodern lens.

# Chapter 1
# Introduction

**marcela polanco, Navid Zamani, and Christina Da Hee Kim**

*Yeki bood, yeki nabood, gheyraz khodah, heech kas nabood.*
*There was someone [bilinguals in the USA], there was no one [bilinguals in MFT],*
*besides God [standard English] there was no one.*

*(Mohammad Ali Jamalzadeh – Persian literature) (Our translation)*

**Abstract** This chapter introduces the contributions of 25 authors who came together as a community to write (for the first time for some) about their bilingual lived experiences. As family therapists and members of various communities, their experiences – illustrated in 18 different languages – shaped 11 chapters on bilingualism, culture, and social justice in family therapy. We introduce their intents for linguistic justice in a field shaped by standard English. We describe the paradoxical complexities of editing a volume that is written mostly in English while advocating for bilingualism. Bilingualism here refers to the complex political, cultural, social, and historical systemic encounters between the standard English family therapy field and the 18 other languages as identified by the authors. Given the current exclusionary effects of English monolingualism on the family therapy field, we include our hopes for the field to adopt anti-racist initiatives from the language perspective.

---

m. polanco (✉)
Marriage and Family Therapy Master's Program & Spanglish/Ingleñol Family Therapy Certificado, San Diego State University, San Diego, CA, USA
e-mail: marcela.polanco@sdsu.edu

N. Zamani
San Diego State University, San Diego, CA, USA

C. D. H. Kim
License to Freedom, El Cajon, CA, USA



m. polanco et al. (eds.), *Bilingualism, Culture, and Social Justice in Family Therapy*, AFTA SpringerBriefs in Family Therapy,
https://doi.org/10.1007/978-3-030-66036-9_1

In the few months that eventually became the inception of this book, we (marcela and Navid) were meeting regularly in Navid's neighborhood in Normal Heights, San Diego, for a morning walk with Navid's 6-month-old, Leila. Normal Heights is a lively residential area pulsing with many hip cafes, gastropubs, bars, and Thai, Mexican, and Ethiopian restaurants. Walking through this community that reflects the cultural diversity of San Diego, we learned about our own respective Fenglish (Farsi-English) (Navid) and Colombian Spanglish (marcela) lives and practices as bilingual family therapists. While the length of our conversations on the importance of editing a book and writing about the cultural and ethical considerations of bilingualism within the prevalent position of monolingual standard English in the marriage and family therapy (MFT) field would quickly lull Leila to sleep in her stroller, the urgency and importance of writing a book of this nature became more palpable to us. Our intent was to advocate for justice in language rights where English reigns in spite of services being delivered by bilingual practitioners to communities that speak languages other than English. Based on our own experiences as instructors, researchers, supervisors, and practitioners in the USA, we had a clear commitment for this book to advance linguistic rights within a monolingual MFT field. Our hopes were that the current and incoming generations of bilingual family therapists would receive the training, acknowledgement, and honoring that protects their linguistic integrity. From our perspective, this would look like a coming together of languages, similar to the way Normal Heights is the coming together of cultural traditions to share space, food, music, and films to create a thriving and lively community. We were hoping that this book would contribute to a linguistic movement in the MFT field whereby the current standard English training curriculums, therapy frameworks, journals, and professional conferences would shift to resemble the multiple languages represented by the streets on which we were walking and the many others around the USA.

## Writing in English to Denounce the Predominance of Standard English

Throughout the preparation of this book during the year 2020, our commitment was impacted by the pivotal moment of the longstanding historical anti-racist movement in the USA, led by Black activists and the Black Lives Matter movement after the killing of many Black community members. We hope for this book to further advance an anti-racist movement calling the MFT field to action toward accountability by monolinguals and bilinguals alike, for the current racial and cultural disparities within the field, in this case, from the vantage point of bilingualism. Part of the call for transformative and sustainable change within the MFT field requires exposing its White supremacist structures, perpetuated in part by the prevalence of standard English monolingualism.

Inevitably, we understood very well that undertaking the editing of this book posed some paradoxical complexities and challenges for us. We wanted to invite contributors to write chapters on the cultural and linguistic considerations of bilingualism that would contest in one way or another the current standing of standard monolingual English in MFT. Yet, we did so with the premise that their chapters had to be written in English. Furthermore, within this contradiction, we wanted to invite practicing family therapists who would tell their stories about their bilingualisms in their training, practice, and/or lives. However, we anticipated that for some, the stories we were inviting them to write may have not been storied before. We understood that, as bilinguals, to discern and understand the skills and knowledge involved in what we are habituated to practice in split seconds, going back and forth across languages, is certainly not an easy task, let alone having to articulate such a highly complex experience and make it tangible to a possible monolingual reader. Yet, we understood that although it is not an easy task, it is an important one. We have been missing out from its immense learning potential – as it is documented in the stories of this book – by not attending to such task given that during our training, and current professional development, opportunities to do so continue to be lacking.

Hence, it was clear to us that our invitation to contribute to this book would have to confront the very same phenomenon we were seeking to address: no previous pedagogical platforms in MFT had been in place for many of us to story and learn from the skills and knowledge embedded within our bilingual lives and practices. The presence of such a platform would not only enrich our practices to better serve bilingual families but would also pay respect to the integrity of our linguistic identities in our positions as therapists. It would provide the opportunity to learn from the unique, complex, and highly sophisticated skills created by and required of living in more than one language in a racialized society that gives prevalence to standard English and English speaking over any other language.

## Writing About Bilingualism and Not About Bilinguals

Our invitation was not only to contributors but to our third editor, Christina DaHee Kim. We met Christina at San Diego State University where we work as instructors and supervisors. The three of us worked together during Christina's training in the Master's program in MFT. For the three of us, it was important that the stories about therapy practice, supervision, training, or everyday life by contributors would be told specifically from the perspective of language and involve some kind of informal analysis of the cultural negotiation of bilingual experiences.

Our clear intent was to keep the discussion as far away as possible from essentializing, hence, racializing communities in relation to the languages spoken, as in the term "Hispanic." The Hispanic identity is a radical example of the construction of a supposedly homogeneous, racialized social category that relates to communities who speak a seeming homogeneous Spanish language. Therefore, we intended for this book to document stories about the intricacies of the languages bilingual family therapists speak in their lives and practices, rather than to tell stories about bilingual family therapists who speak other than standard English language. For example, in relation to the term Hispanic, the emphasis would be on the implications of speaking Spanish in the USA and not on Hispanics who speak Spanish in the USA. This is a subtle but radical shift in perspective. Our interest was to expose the institutional, academic, professional, governmental, or other structures and policies that regulate and implement exclusionary practices against bilingualism with material implications in the lives of family therapists in the USA. But we had no interest in the stories of this book claiming to speak for and in the absence of others who speak similar languages in homogeneous ways. We radically stand in opposition to this sort of multicultural politics of representation of communities. We hoped that the 6 chapters in this book (out of 12) by family therapists who locate their lives, practices, and/or identity with various Spanish languages illustrate this by discounting a homogenous, standard version of the Spanish language or Spanish speakers.

## Becoming Bilingual Authors and Editors Within the English Language

Implicit within our invitation to contributors in this book was the matter of becoming authors. We intentionally included folxs who had not published their work before. The daunting task at times of becoming authors within the context of the US publishing industry for the first time was not something some had considered before. We found it important to highlight the consideration of becoming authors as bilingual therapists since we believe that it also pertains to the position that standard English has in the field. A brief look at the available literature in family therapy and required reading material lists in course syllabi would quickly reveal whose work gets published and whose is not. It seems quite apparent to us whose languages, therefore family therapists, continue to be excluded from the body of work in MFT.

The knowledge production in the field continues to be in the single hands of standard English no matter the languages spoken by those whose work gets published and who consume and practice it in English or other languages. Those of us who are bilinguals with skills to write in either language, and have a platform to publish, default to English as the language that shapes our thinking and body of work. We believe this to be shaped by the politics of a knowledge machine (e.g., textbooks, publishers, universities, professional organizations, etc.) that holds global power drawn from a history of imperialism and colonialism, defaulting necessarily to infiltrate this world through the language of the colonizer.

Moreover, the MFT literature that is available in non-English languages is in its majority a translation of standard English written texts. While it is important that these texts are made available in non-English languages, the translated frameworks remain shaped by the epistemological and ontological foundations that are structured by the perspectives of the original standard English texts. While this book is also primarily written in English, the perspectives do come from various epistemological linguistic vantage points.

As first-time book editors, from our Colombian Spanglish (marcela), Fenglish (Navid), and Konglish (Korean-English) (Christina) perspectives, we grappled with the ongoing tensions between writing in the language whose prevalence we sought to challenge. We attempted to promote a space for authors to articulate the symbolisms, cultural variations, and vocabularies that honor the identities of non-English languages we invited them to write about. And, on the contrary, we also promoted what we believed to be a somewhat standard organization of standard English writing and grammar. We navigated the tension of these two opposing perspectives with the gracious support of the community of contributors.

## The Community of Contributors: Writing During the COVID-19 Pandemic

Twenty-five contributors came together. We had a previous relationship with them through our work and communities and shared, in our own particular ways, aspects of an anti-racist bilingual advocacy stance. Their ideas shaped 11 chapters containing short stories on bilingualism, culture, and social justice in family therapy. Bilingualism, in the 11 chapters, included 18 languages identified by the authors: Black Talk/Ebonics/Slang, Farsi, Fenglish, Arabic, Italian, Cantonese Chinese, South Korean, Mandarin Chinese, Vietnamese, Spanish, Chilean Spanish, Mexican Spanish, Colombian Spanglish, Madrileño Spanish, Spanglish, Pocho Spanish, Colloquial Spanish, and English. Most of the contributors are family therapists local to San Diego. We met one way or another through our different affiliations with San Diego State University. marcela knew Carlos A. Ramos, Jimena Castro, and Joseph Alvaro Guerrero from their mutual connection with Our Lady of the Lake University in San Antonio, Texas.

During the preparation of the chapters, we held monthly collective meetings online to have conversations about our interests, work, and experiences with bilingualism as family therapists. And we met with various authors to exchange ideas with the intent to support their writing. The editing and writing of this book took place in great part during the COVID pandemic and the anti-racist national and global unrest that was ignited by the killing of George Floyd at the hands of police officers on May 25, 2020. All of us sustained a shared commitment to this project in spite of the rapid restructuring of our lives under a quarantine and rightful protests against anti-Blackness and structural racism. Throughout this experience, our understanding on our own bilingualities was transformed from what we learned from each contributor's stories.

## The Contributor's Stories We Learned

The rich description of Thien's home in California at the beginning of Cho, Pham, and Chung's chapter brought to life a Vietnamese "feel" and "smell" that set an aesthetic context for their discussion on intersecting linguistic considerations. This imagery opens the book. It invited us to "take our shoes off" as we entered into a sort of migration of languages throughout the stories in the various chapters. While the chapters were written in English, as X, Chau, Hogan, and polanco warned us, they were written without entirely leaving their non-standard English languages behind. This provided us with an opportunity to come across familiar and unfamiliar languages, thus at times tripping over unfamiliar vocabularies when authors intentionally did not translate their vocabularies for us into standard English. This came to be the quality of an ongoing reminder that engaging language differences implicates an inter-linguistic encounter.

In the first four chapters of the book, through the particular vantage points of Asian languages (Cho, Pham, and Chung), Borderland Spanglish (X, Chau, Hogan, and polanco), Italian (Guidarelli), and Talking Black/Ebonics (Vaughn and Mosley), contributors storied the particular linguistic considerations of living, training, doing therapy, and relating professionally in standard English, White Talk (Vaughn and Mosley), and their non-standard English languages. Their stories situated language in bilingualism as what Guidarelli described in *la questione della lingua*, a matter of being another person when speaking in another language. Guidarelli borrowed from the Second Language Acquisition literature to embody the symbolic power of language arguing that languages create realities, hence identities.

In the same line and from the vantage point of the authors' Cantonese Chinese, South Korean, Mandarin Chinese, Vietnamese, and Spanish, Cho, Pham, and Chung addressed the discussion of linguistic identities through their training and practice. Having experienced their family therapy training as an act of socialization into what they called a "Therapy Speak" in standard English, they storied how they grappled with lacking not only confidence but linguistic knowledge to practice in their Asian languages. While they argued that being able to practice in non-English languages is not only a matter of language proficiency, later, Ocampo-Giancola, Alvarez, and Murga, when storing their experiences navigating Pocho Spanish, Spanglish, and Spanish, advocated for the need of training support for language proficiency in order to practice in their Spanish. They argued that practicing in their Spanish, hence to engage *corazón*/heart in their work, similar to Cho, Pham, and Chung, the development of a diverse set of linguistic skills is required. They storied their journey as three Mexican first-generation bilingual (Pocho Spanish, Spanish, and Spanglish speakers) clinicians becoming family therapists enduring anti-immigration sentiments and linguistic discrimination. Like Vaughn and Mosley's Black Talk perspective and Zamani and Zamani's *amianeh* (slang) Farsi, they also challenged the discourse of languages that are non-standard English as "less educated."

X, Chau, Hogan, and polanco problematized translation as a seamless switch across languages and accents and into the borderlands. For them, it involves a kind of trafficking and smuggling of languages across inhospitable linguistic borders. This is so as to discover a new aesthetical linguistic existence “through syntax, imagery, evocation, and metaphor” not otherwise possible in English. Furthermore, from a different linguistic location (like Vaughn and Mosley’s Talking Black bilingualism) X, Chau, Hogan, and polanco questioned the effects of standard English in the professionalization and whitening of their lives and practices. Vaughn and Mosley had a conversation among themselves, *keepin’ it real* to *speakin’* to rebel against the inferiorization of Black Talk. They revealed to us the effects of internal colonization endured by Black family therapists as the embodiment of a linguistic code switching between Black and White Talk when in professional conversations with non-Black people.

Zamani and Zamani (Farsi and Fenglish); Ramos, Castro, and Guerrero Velez (Spanish); and Ramirez Ibarra’s (Spanish) chapters storied their therapy practices through the particularities of their non-English vantage points. In their work with Farsi-speaking clients and their Fenglish language, Zamani and Zamani connect their narrative therapy practices. Within the historical and political contexts of Farsi, and the cultural considerations of relating in Farsi, they expanded narrative therapy practices yet maintaining fidelity to its ethical tenets. They advocated for politics of imperfection when attempting to adopt Fenglish language in therapy while embodying the experience of the *rooh* (spirit).

Ramos, Castro, and Guerrero Velez staged their stories about their practice in Spanish in Cervantes’s classic Spanish novel, *Don Quijote de la Mancha*. They drew from the novelistic oral traditions of their Spanish depicted in *Don Quijote* to illustrate what they described as a Latinx practice of *chismorreo*/gossiping. This is as a dialogical process they described as particular to their Spanish language. They shared stories of their therapy sessions in Spanish through *chismorreo* to engage non-linearly the senses, imagination, fascination, and novelty. Nidya Ramirez’s stories also address considerations of conducting therapeutic conversations in Spanish with Latinx communities; however she does through a critique toward the English-based trauma narratives that are translated and transferred into her psychotherapy in Spanish. She highlighted the particular cultural variations in Spanish from the Latinx clients she works with that are embedded in unique vocabularies that are quite distinct from the English narratives of trauma.

Lugo storied her journey of becoming a Spanglish-English supervisor in response to the lack of bilingual training support during her own formation as a family therapist. She offered a description of the complexities of supporting the training of Spanish-English trainees who are being perceived as favored against trainees who are speakers of other non-English languages. She also described the various adaptations of clinical practice into Spanish in her supervision. In line with the critique Lugo and others offer to the lack of training support to bilinguals in family therapy, Chau, Estrella, Guerrieri, and O’Sullivan situate their critique from their Chilean, Mexican, and Colombian Spanish. They storied the development of their own community of support they affectionately called *Las Comadres*. They shared clinical developments that emerged from their *comadres'* community while grappling with their untranslatable English family therapy training and Spanish. They turned to their linguistic street-cred to articulate practices of their own, where they traffic their English and Spanish in a way that they argue is not welcome in academic or professional settings. Therefore, they called their practice *terapia de la calle*, or street therapy, where they speak *palabras de a centavo*, or colloquial Spanish, that includes their familiar and "warm" vocabularies.

Stories of the English and Arabic languages that are teamed up in a domestic violence intervention program by Rogers, Darbi, and Leverman close the book. Their work took us to reminisce about our pre-COVID morning walks with Leila through the intercultural streets of Normal Heights. They offered an account of a coming together of languages, English and Arabic, in a team of responders to and sufferers from the effects of violence within Middle Eastern families to share space and stories. They storied their experiences of doing therapy with an interpreter as a means to create language communities through building relational bridges within a client-interpreter-and-therapist team.

## As We Move Forward…

We hope that you, the reader, can stroll through this book in the ways we strolled through our neighborhoods in San Diego. While doing so, we hope that you capture from the contributors' stories an appreciation for the multiple linguistic experiences, recognizing their broader complexities situated in the historical, social, and political contexts of life. While the important therapy work captured here is primarily occurring in our local community, San Diego, California, and also in San Antonio, Texas, we are aware that many others, in various regions of the USA, are also doing critical bilingual and polylingual work although hidden in plain sight. We hope they feel a similar sense of urgency in contributing to this body of literature. Therefore, it is our hope that this book serves as an invitation to bilingual family therapists to consider points of connection as well as points of departure from the ideas and experiences captured here, so they also make their stories available to monolingual and polylingual family therapists. As therapy continues to expand beyond the edges of the standard English language, we rely on bilinguals' voices and experiences to continue to complexify areas of inquiry in family therapy across multiple languages. This is so that no longer we are put in the position to have to simplify the descriptions of our multilingual practices when choosing to privilege the current "Englished" monolingual family therapy field so our practices can fit in.

# Chapter 2
# Intersections of Asian Identity, Languages, and Professional Education: Where the Personal and Professional Intimately Collide

**Wonyoung L. Cho, Thien T. Pham, and Diana K. Chung**

**Abstract** Despite the continuing trend of diversifying ethnic, cultural, and linguistic identities of systemic therapy students and clinicians in the United States, there is still a dearth of research and literature in the areas of multilingual clinician education and practice. This gap in research and resources leaves many students and practitioners without much guidance as they serve marginalized, non-English-speaking communities who are relatively unfamiliar with the culture of therapy. In this chapter, three multilingual Asian American practitioners (Chinese American, Korean American, and Vietnamese American) share anecdotes from the beginning stages of their careers learning to serve communities in their various non-English and heritage languages. Through our personal experiences, we will discuss the intersection of language(s), personal and professional identities, and Asian American experience as it relates to clinical practice and education.

The homes of my (Thien) immigrant clients in California closely resembled my childhood home. Couches from the 1980s, snacks and dried goods spilling from the kitchen counter and tables, a rice cooker and large pots for soup, countless to-go containers washed and stored for future uses, and a fridge overflowing with fresh meats and vegetables. Knick knacks and Costco™ bulk items coexist throughout the house as if to show abundance and frugality at the same time. There is often a

W. L. Cho (✉)
Marriage, Couples, and Family Therapy, Lewis & Clark Graduate School of Education and Counseling, Portland, OR, USA

Lewis & Clark College, Portland, OR, USA
e-mail: wonyoungcho@lclark.edu

T. T. Pham
Private Practice, San Francisco, CA, USA

D. K. Chung
Community Health and Private Practice, Alhambra, CA, USA



m. polanco et al. (eds.), *Bilingualism, Culture, and Social Justice in Family Therapy*, AFTA SpringerBriefs in Family Therapy,
https://doi.org/10.1007/978-3-030-66036-9_2

stew, soup, or both on the stove. The smell of fish sauce is potent, but familiar. Somewhere in the living room, there is some Vietnamese shell acrylic art of horses, a calendar from the local Vietnamese dentist or doctor, and a TV that is probably too old for this decade. The kitchen table is decorated with plastic lining with bright patterns and a bowl of fresh fruit readily available. Nothing matches, as most of these items were gifted or thrifted. In this space, I am often reminded of my own childhood and the struggles of trying to make a foreign place feel like home.

When entering the home, I instinctively remember to take my shoes off. I would take a quick scan and rank people from oldest to youngest and be ready to bow and use appropriate titles to acknowledge and pay respect to the eldest member, which is often a grandparent. Even though I was only in my mid-20s at this time, parents would greet me with a kinship term[1] that would surpass my perceived age. In Vietnam, there's a culture of overestimating someone's kinship term to show respect and humility. While the parents would normally call me *em* or *con*, a title given to someone who is generally younger and less experienced in life, I'm often given the title *chị* or *cô* due to the perceived authority I have as a trained professional. I chose early on to keep age-appropriate kinship terms out of my own discomfort of appearing more authoritative. This was both a professional and personal choice.

As 1.5- and second-generation immigrants[2] ourselves, we (the authors of this chapter) instinctively relate to the intimate experiences of our own childhood and familial relationships when navigating these cultural and personal spaces of our clients as mental health clinicians. According to the 2011 Census data, 76.7% of households identifying as only Asian in the United States spoke a language other than English at home (Ryan 2013). This number is projected to rise if the data accounted for families with more than one ethnic or racial identity. Therapists who are heritage language[3] speakers, bilingual, and/or multilingual may be more likely to be employed to provide mental health services for these families whose primary language is not English. In other words, therapists who are identified as hyphenated Americans (e.g., Chinese American, Korean American, Vietnamese American) and have grown up with a non-English language in their homes are often expected to meet the needs of families within their own racial and ethnic communities. Yet, there is very little to no research and literature on the education and clinical practices of these multilingual clinicians. There is further dearth of research and

[1] Kinship terms are titles used to identify specific relationships between members of the same community.

[2] The term "first-generation" is often used to identify those who immigrated to the United States in their adulthood, after they have been socialized in another country. "Second-generation" is used to identify those who are born in the United States to first-generation parents. Thus, "1.5-generation" is often used to identify those in between – people who immigrated to the United States earlier in their lives and are socialized in both cultures.

[3] Heritage language specifically refers to language that is associated with one's ethnicity, homes, and family that is not used outside the home by the host culture as the dominant language (Lee 2013).

literature on the multilingual experiences of Asian American clinicians serving the Asian immigrant and Asian American communities.

The authors of this chapter, like many other Asian Americans and immigrants who have come before us, are no strangers to stepping into a Eurocentric monolingual context and carving out third spaces that retain remnants of our heritage. We are licensed marriage and family therapists (MFT) who speak more than one language in our daily lives and have served communities whose primary language is not English. Between the three authors of this chapter, many languages are represented: Cantonese Chinese, South Korean, Mandarin Chinese, Spanish, and Vietnamese. Wonyoung is a fully bilingual Korean American, who was born in South Korea and came to the United States when she was 9 years old. Thien was born in Vietnam and immigrated to California at age nine. Diana identifies as a Chinese American born in the United States. All of our proficiencies in our various languages have fluctuated over the course of our lives.

## Becoming a Professional

We (the authors of this chapter) became therapists together. We attended the same marriage and family therapy program, which was immersed in poststructural and social constructionist thought at the time (e.g., Monk et al. 2008; Burr 2003). Our graduate education was in English: we learned law and ethics in English, explored theories of practice in English, and role-played in English. Our specialist language, a particular "way with words" (p. 23, Gee 2014) used by particular groups of people, was also limited to English. At the same time, due to the strong social constructionist influence in our training, we were encouraged to ask for the meanings of words that the clients, colleagues, and professionals used rather than assume that the way we understood a word was the same way others understood it. For me (Wonyoung), this critical stance on language and languaging was foundational in doing the work of bridging between languages in my clinical practice.

In some ways, asking for meaning and definitions felt familiar. There was something in my lived experiences as a language broker (McQuillan and Tse 1995, as cited in Shen et al. 2014) in my family and struggling to translate back and forth between languages that confirmed this need to be suspicious of assumed meanings of words. Over time and with accruing clinical experiences, I began to peel back the layers of language within the English language as I learned how to practice: the colloquial, the academic, the mental health expert, and a blend of the three that emerged specifically in therapeutic contexts. We will refer to this unique blend of the colloquial, academic, and specialist social languages as "Therapy Speak."

The socialization into Therapy Speak was gradual and almost undetectable. It began to creep into our everyday language, and our friends outside of the mental health field would notice we started talking differently. I (Diana) recall enlightened conversations with other marriage and family therapy students in which we would speak diagnosis, acronyms, and about where we *manifested emotions somatically*.

Therapy Speak was the new normal, and like any common identity of shared language speakers, I felt a part of the exclusive club of therapists reveling in a sense of competence. As a vulnerable therapist, green with inexperience, it felt safe to hide behind the guise of our new therapy vernacular.

Now as a clinical supervisor of bilingual therapy students, I see this familiar pattern played out by prospective candidates in both English and Spanish. I am audience to performances of elevated therapy jargon of English words conveying modern Anglo and Eurocentric concepts to be disseminated in the family language of our clients. These ideas remain poorly translated on mental health questionnaires in non-English languages, leaving clients at a loss about how to answer them, further creating distance between client and therapist. It has taken time to deconstruct Therapy Speak in English and Spanish to reconnect with the language, beliefs, and spirit of client work in minority populations. I reflect on a powerful YouTube video by a Vietnamese American public figure speaking about her family's experience of abuse and subsequent mental health issues (Mai 2019). She described depression and anxiety stemming from traumas as "family curses," which feel much more familiar and digestible than *intergenerational trauma*. It is important to become competent in Therapy Speak and then unlearn it by privileging the language of our clients.

## Colliding with the Personal

When initially presented with an opportunity to do therapy in another language, several key memories of visits to my mother's birth city of Hong Kong and struggles of stumbling over my (Diana) words came to the surface, making me feel small. I stood out so much there and got comments about how American I dressed and spoke. Needless to say, I wasn't exactly feeling confident and empowered to take on the task of learning how to do therapy in Cantonese. At that point in my career, I was learning the artful concepts of therapy for the first time and not sure if I was up to the task to endure the process in two languages and cultures.

Nonetheless, I began researching what it would take to become a bilingual Cantonese therapist for several reasons – to give back to my community, for family pride, and because maybe I could actually do it. I didn't even know if Cantonese people went to therapy; I certainly didn't know of any. I consulted with my mom on the phone and during visits home. She taught me the phrases for mental health experiences like depression and anxiety. She taught me how to say "confidentiality" the formal way – (機密) *gei mut*. After evaluating the context of how this word was to be used in therapy, she then explained to me the way a typical layperson would actually understand, (保密) *bo mut*, meaning "to protect secrets."

Despite my efforts to connect to this local knowledge and linguistically "grow up" enough to play the role of therapist, it was no match for the semi-paved road ahead of me to develop as a Spanish-speaking therapist. Unlike in my heritage language of Cantonese, I have built up to graduate-level education in Spanish and have immersed myself in the language when going to school abroad. Contrary to feeling exposed and vulnerable at times in Cantonese, Spanish makes me feel grown-up and powerful. I debated my grade with a pompous professor, negotiated a rate for my English tutoring side-hustle, and broke a lease on a shady apartment in Madrid. *Yo me puedo defender con la lengua.* For me, Spanish doesn't come with cultural and linguistic expectations from other speakers like Cantonese does and subsequently doesn't carry the disappointment and struggle.

Conducting therapy as an outsider in predominantly Latinx communities has resulted in a dance of navigating culture, language, and the negotiation of knowledge. Academic Spanish allows access to provide mental health services to Hispanic families. However, gaining the acceptance and cooperation of parents in therapy with a non-Latinx therapist requires an additional level of joining for which Therapy Speak and elevated Spanish are not as helpful. I've acquired vocabulary of colloquial and anglicized words[4] from my clients that are specific to the community to be able to relate. Drawing from experiences of my Chinese identity and patchwork language ability, I empathize with the parents and children I work with who can't seem to find a mutual tongue. Therapy becomes a joint effort in stitching together the client's experiences and our mutual knowledge to create meaning.

## Reintegrating Our Whole Selves: Intersection of Language, Culture, and Identity

Language is a tool and a medium with which we communicate and transmit information, embedded with culturally specific ideologies and discourses (Fairclough 2013). It is also integral to the performance of our own identities and communicating who we are to others, the audience(s) in our lives (Gee 2014). Thus, conducting therapeutic conversations in a non-English language requires more than simple language proficiency. Language proficiency gives the speaker flexibility in the way they may shape or design the language to convey meanings, but it does not always equate to having the social, historical, and cultural knowledge needed to shape the language artfully for therapeutic effect. This distinction is crucial in therapeutic contexts, because language is not just about communicating content and meaning. Language shapes the experiences of our clients in therapeutic contexts. Language is also integral to performing our identities and profession as a therapist.

With artful languaging, we become a younger sister, an older brother, a child, a parent, a mentor, a supervisor, a colleague, or a friend. The way we speak to our romantic partner is different from the way we would speak to a coworker in a professional setting or a stranger we have met for the first time. Living in the United States where English dominates a good portion of our lives and socialization, we often have varied experiences of diverse relationships using the English language.

---

[4] Anglicisms are originally English words that are modified and incorporated into other languages.

Standard English is polished and used in our education systems, casual English is spoken in social contexts when we are out with our friends, and a hybrid language of our heritage language and English (e.g., Spanglish, Konglish) is spoken when we are with our close family and friends within our cultural groups. All of us, monolingual, bilingual, and multilingual speakers living in the United States often have experiences of fluidly moving between these relationships and adjusting our languaging within English accordingly.

In contrast with the diverse relationships and social performances based in English, the non-English languages in our lives are often limited within the confines of our personal and intimate relationships. For example, most of my (Wonyoung) Korean language use since moving to the United States has been limited to my family life. Korean speakers in the United States who are 1.5- and second-generation immigrants often associate the Korean language with intimate and immediate experiences of their families of origin (e.g., Kang 2013). Thus, the self that is being conjured and performed in this Korean language is often limited to that of a child relating to their parents, grandparents, and elders in the community. Oftentimes, this particular style of languaging is the only kind of Korean languaging that the Korean heritage language speakers are familiar with in the United States.

Becoming a professional and conducting therapeutic conversations in my heritage language of Korean is much more than becoming proficient in mental health terminologies. I had to start with the languaging I was familiar with as a child in relations to my parents and elders in my community. I asked my parents for words and became their young daughter again, rather than the independent adult child who did not need her parents anymore. Then I had to incorporate other parts of my Korean language self that seemed far from professional and almost inappropriate to conjure up in therapeutic spaces. I pulled from the casual Konglish I spoke with my friends into my therapeutic conversations. I imagined my Korean self more complexly and broadly, beyond the family relationships and mimicking some of the languaging and mannerisms of professionals I saw in Korean television dramas. I incorporated what I learned about relationships from lyrics of K-pop songs from my angsty teenage years. I had to reintegrate my whole self into this role of the Korean-speaking therapist, including who I was casually on my off-time when I am not a therapist.

I do not mean that I relate to clients as a child or an angsty teenager or a character from a Korean drama. I also do not mean that I am not professional and knowledgeable as a therapist. I had to be multifaceted in my Korean, the way I am multifaceted in my English. This required me to develop myself complexly in Korean, the same way I have developed myself complexly in English. This required more than Korean language proficiency: it required deeper self-of-the-therapist work. It required revisiting the relationships within my family and working out relational traumas I had experienced from my community in my heritage language. It required me to reach out to the laypeople in my community for words and language. It required me to be humble in my professional stance and hold what my community knew about mental health in equal value to what I had learned in my graduate training. And more than anything, it inspired a more complex development of my own self in my heritage language.

Becoming a multilingual therapist and practicing in a non-English language are more than speaking another language. It means that we are involved in a much more complex process of negotiating identities, experiences, and cultures. It is an uncharted territory of our professional development. And yet, we have learned from our lived immigrant experiences what it means to be resourceful, to collect wisdom from our own communities, and to seek mentoring through personal channels. We (the authors of this chapter) have also learned that we need each other. It is vital to forge our own village of multilingual and multicultural colleagues to witness the complexity and importance of our experience as therapists. We share our anecdotes and experiences, as "older sisters" who have foraged our own resources in working with clients who often are members of our own community. We also humbly recognize that we are not the only ones who have walked this road, as there are many mentors and trailblazers who have journeyed ahead of us and have taught us what we know. As we share and document our learnings, we are hopeful that it will be a stepping stone for those who will join us and follow after us in articulating what we inherently know from our lived experiences to shape how to better serve our non-English-speaking communities.

## References


Burr, V. (2003). *Social constructionism* (2nd ed.). London; New York: Routledge.

Fairclough, N. (2013). Language and ideology. In N. Fairclough (Ed.), *Critical discourse analysis: The critical study of language* (2nd ed., pp. 56–68). England: Routledge.

Gee, J. P. (2014). Introduction. In J. P. Gee (Ed.), *An introduction to discourse analysis: Theory and method* (4th ed., pp. 2–15). London: Routledge.

Kang, H. S. (2013). Korean American college students' language practices and identity positioning: "Not Korean, but not American.". *Journal of Language, Identity & Education, 12*(4), 248–261. https://doi.org/10.1080/15348458.2013.818473.

Lee, B. Y. (2013). Heritage language maintenance and cultural identity formation: The case of Korean immigrant parents and their children in the USA. *Early Child Development and Care, 183*(11), 1576–1588. https://doi.org/10.1080/03004430.2012.741125.

Mai, J. (2019, October 17). *My mom opens up about her childhood trauma* [Video]. YouTube. https://www.youtube.com/watch?v=Oikugkvy1HE

Monk, G., Winslade, J., & Sinclair, S. L. (2008). *New horizons in multicultural counseling*. Los Angeles: Sage Publications.

Ryan, C. (2013). Language use in the United States: 2011. *American Community Survey Reports*. Retrieved from https://www.census.gov/library/publications/2013/acs/acs-22.html

Shen, Y., Kim, S. Y., Wang, Y., & Chao, R. K. (2014). Language brokering and adjustment among Chinese and Korean American adolescents: A moderated mediation model of perceived maternal sacrifice, respect for the mother, and mother–child open communication. *Asian American Journal of Psychology, 5*(2), 86–95. https://doi.org/10.1037/a0035203.

# Chapter 3
# Storying the Aesthetics of *Nuestras* Linguistic Borderlands: A Tapestry *de* Solidarity

**Tisha X, Mu-Lan Chau, Lorraine Hogan, and marcela polanco**

**Abstract** As bilingual marriage and family therapists (MFTs), here we attempt to describe our aesthetic linguistic borderlands as a new place where we exist at the juncture of our English and Spanish. We tell our stories of untranslatability; woven in a narrative tapestry of threads made of our experiences of migrating back and forth across the linguistic, geo-socio-political, and historical borders of English and *Español*. We share experiences of exclusion, discrimination, and racism against our accents and Spanglish borderland languages. We intend to summon the English-configured MFT field to meet us at the border of their monolingual wall and see past it, into a different world of existence, through syntax, imagery, evocation, and metaphor. We challenge Eurocentric foundations that situate English as the dominant way to language the world and therapy. Intentionally – and ironically – we write about our experiences in English, but without entirely leaving the aesthetics of our Spanish behind.

---

We want to give special recognition to our colleagues Marissa Barajas, Shinyung Oh, Kimberly Ayres, Candea Mosley, Brittney Romine, and David Epston for their very important contributions to this chapter. Their threads are also woven into this tapestry.

---

Tisha X (✉) · M.-L. Chau
Associate Marriage and Family Therapist, Riverside, CA, USA

L. Hogan
Marriage and Family Therapist, San Diego, CA, USA

m. polanco
Marriage and Family Therapy Master's Program & Spanglish/Ingleñol Family Therapy Certificado, San Diego State University, San Diego, CA, USA

 
m. polanco et al. (eds.), *Bilingualism, Culture, and Social Justice in Family Therapy*, AFTA SpringerBriefs in Family Therapy,
https://doi.org/10.1007/978-3-030-66036-9_3

This chapter is a tapestry of linguistic solidarity[1] woven with the threads of our stories as Spanish- and Spanglish-speaking therapists in San Diego, United States. Our tapestry was made in response to the failure of the marriage and family therapy (MFT) field to recognize and be accountable to multilingual practitioners and communities. Our stories and reflections embroidered in this tapestry summon the unique struggles of bilingual MFTs. We attempt to describe our aesthetic linguistic borderlands, a new linguistic place where we exist at the juncture of our English and Spanish, creating a "bastard language...not approved by any society" (Anzaldua 1999, p. 21). As we describe our borderland experience in relation to language, we also portray our historical, social, and political realities.[2]

Our heritages are rooted linguistically in our borderlands' storytelling traditions that only recently began to intentionally enter our MFT practices. Here we attempt to story what we are learning as we arrive at our borderlands. We tell of the untranslatability between Spanish and English when migrating back and forth across its linguistic, geo-socio-political, and historical borders. We share experiences of discrimination and racism against our accents and Spanglish borderland language in our personal and professional lives. We bear the responsibility of legitimizing our bilingual immigrant identities and/or heritages within a Eurocentric academic institution that has eradicated the existence of our Spanish, deeming them inferior to English.

Though efforts have been made to explore social justice and multiculturalism in the MFT field, we find ourselves poorly represented and prepared to maintain the integrity of our linguistic heritages within a monolingual paradigm. These isolating and devastating experiences mirror the historical, political, and social realities that impact not only the therapists but oftentimes the communities we serve. In response, we sought camaraderie among Spanish and Spanglish speakers who were also reckoning with a field largely founded and built for English speakers. Together we have come to resist the monolingualism that unintentionally renders our linguistic identities illegitimate.

The purpose of our tapestry is to invite the English-configured MFT field to meet us at the border of their monolingualism and to see past the wall into a different world of syntax, imagery, evocation, and metaphor. We challenge Eurocentric foundations that situate English as the dominant way to understand the world and lead therapy. Intentionally – and ironically – we write about our experiences in English but without entirely leaving each of our Spanish behind. We do this with the hope that by entrusting our stories to this field, it will open the borders of monolingual practices and welcome our existence alongside the current English monopoly in marriage and family therapy. Respectively, we are four women who have

---

[1]We are guided by politics of solidarity from a decolonizing perspective founded on an interest in creating alliances of mutual recognition, accountability, and respect across differences. See Mohanty (2003).

[2]We subscribe to a Foucauldian poststructural view of language as a constitutive discourse of life that is not separated but configured within its historical, social, cultural, and political contexts of power. See Foucault (1972).

determined our lives from the vantage points of our experiences as: a Colombiana Spanglish-speaking immigrant and MFT educator and three MFT trainees – a first-generation borderland Xicana who speaks Spanish she inherited from Oaxaca, Mexico, and Spanglish birthed in San Diego, California; a Chilean immigrant; and a biracial Spanish and Black American immigrant – whose stories are as follows. We met in 2018 when we became part of the MFT master's program at San Diego State University (SDSU).

In writing this chapter, we, as members of SDSU, seek to respect and honor the Kumeyaay, Yuman-speaking people, the original guardians of the land where SDSU currently resides. We acknowledge the ongoing replications of colonial structures represented in a Western university training program on indigenous land. We also want to honor and pay our respects to the Zapotecs, Mapuches, Africans, Musicas, and Campesinxs of our respective lands and heritages in the Americas. From our ancestors, we learn that storytelling is an oral tradition that weaves together their histories in a tapestry that protects, honors, and keeps alive the integrity of their existences. Thus, our stories here seek to join a history etched in the soil of generations of resistance against the centrism of Western languages and institutions perpetuated by colonial power. Guided by ancestral traditions, we storytell our struggles to protect and preserve the legitimacy and integrity of our linguistic existence in Spanish, Spanglish, and English as MFTs.

## Tisha: *Una Coyote de Lenguaje* – A Language Trafficker

As a first-generation Xicana who grew up a few miles north of *la frontera*, the border wall that separates Tijuana, Mexico *de* San Diego, United States, I know all too well the kinds of separations borders create. As a bilingual therapist I found my work to be another casualty of this separation. On one side of *el* wall were linguistic knowledge native to my academic English about how to be a therapist. On the other was an embroidery of linguistic knowledge indigenous to *mi Español*, hand-woven by colorful Oaxacan threads of *cultura*.

As a bilingual therapist I needed to find a way to address this separation. Since my English had never been stopped, questioned, or searched at any checkpoint, it was the first to venture across the linguistic border. Although my English expected to cross without any problems, surprisingly, when it set foot on foreign soil during my first Spanish session, it became evident it would not be able to survive the journey intact. Thus, crossing *la frontera* became the responsibility of *mi Español*, but every time it tried to cross via a legal point of entry, it would get stopped by *la migra por no tener papeles*. Therefore, like countless others before me, and many more to come after, I knew that the only chance it had to make it across the border would require me to become a *coyote de lenguaje*, a language trafficker, tasked with finding safe passage for *mi Español* into my English. However, *mi Español* never made it past *el cerro*, the desert of translation, as it was captured by *la migra*, treated as a criminal, and held in a detention center indefinitely, as it was perceived to be smuggling in inferior linguistic and cultural contraband that threatened proper and professional English practices.

As a *coyote* for *mi Español*, I took countless trips across the desert of translation in an attempt to professionalize my Spanish practice by acculturating it into English. However, these trips instead reflected in my practice when having to do things like think in Spanish and speak in English while justifying to my non-Spanish-speaking supervisor what I had done in session for the past 50 minutes – well more like an hour, as Spanish sessions tend to run a bit later because time is conceptualized differently *en Español*. My heart-wrenching journeys across the desert made me realize that my translations were an attempt to unweave my Spanish embroidery and reweave it with threads of English culture, which was an act of linguistic violence and thus ethnocide.

*Así que no hubo de otra*, there was no other way, but to realize that *mi Español* could not cross *la frontera* and be translated into English therapeutic existence. At that moment, my Spanish practice began existing *en mi Español* as I began to think, feel, listen, and speak in my borderland Xicana dialect. That was when knowing how to be a therapist *en mi Español* stopped being policed by English theories written in books and instead became an artisanship of relationality with the families I sat with in sessions. With them by my side, we were now free to co-create what it meant for us to relate in our linguistic territories. My conversations with Spanish-speaking families made me question the unquestionable: my dependence on English to outline the borders of what could be deemed as therapeutic. For the first time, I had the option to exist in a world where being a borderland *terapista* was not defined by the atrocities that occur *en la pinche frontera* – the fucking border wall.

## Mu-Lan: Holding onto My *Chilenismos* Through My Intuition

Born and raised *Chilena*, I have known Chinese, Mestiza, Mapuche, and Spaniard roots as well as others that have been lost throughout generations. Due to the different cultures I was raised in throughout my life, I relate to the feeling of being positioned in different imaginary borderlands. This imaginary *fronteras* became more evident when I came to pursue my studies in the United States, where for the first time, I felt embedded in my Chilean roots. This whole process of my MFT training made me question where I should stand, particularly given the background of my different cultures. Interestingly, trying to convey my experience as a Spanglish/bilingual therapist made me feel as confused and lost as practicing in Spanish while getting trained in English. This process has been based purely on intuition, honoring my *tierra* and my ancestors, by importing my knowledge along with my community's experiences. How could I provide therapy in Spanish if I have little to nothing *para agarrarme* (to hold on)? I was even told – by a Spanglish-speaking supervisor – that doing therapy in Spanish should not be a struggle, since it is just translating. Well, it is not. While navigating my MFT journey, I felt I was sailing in harsh and choppy waters, perhaps not unlike my Chinese ancestors in the early 1900s who sailed across the Pacific before finally coming ashore in Chile and learning to live in a different country without knowing the language.

As I sat with the first client I worked with in Spanish, my body felt as if I woke up to the same 8.7 magnitude earthquake that struck Chile in 2010. My Chilean words were shaking, crumbling, and fragmented to the extent that I was not able to craft inquiries in my mother tongue. *¿Pero cómo*, shouldn't this go smoother? – as if it was just a matter of translation. I tried, unsuccessfully, to seek refuge in the theoretical structures of my MFT training in English. However, I was unable to convey in Spanish the ideas that I would have otherwise had in English. But, how? *¡Es* my mother tongue! I felt I was doing something wrong. My heart grew heavy as I was at a loss and on my own.

I tried translating standard English checklists into Spanish, among other things, but I eventually realized that my Spanish sessions were in constant comparison with my English sessions. Drained of energy, I let my intuition – informed by my ancestors and acquired knowledge – guide me away from my English training as it had not provided me with instructions to navigate my bilingual practice.

My intuition steered me toward finding a community of other Spanish-speaking therapists who were also navigating, questioning, and wondering about their bilingual practices. No longer on my own, I began to bring back *mis* cultural linguistics *chilenismos* that had gotten lost on the therapeutic land. This community embraced and helped me to trust myself and let my creativity engage in a wonderland with all sorts of symbolisms and *dichos* that were evoked in sessions. As a bilingual therapist, I have had to reconnect and embrace my *chilenismos* to *agarrarlos* while traversing the imaginary territories of my Spanish and English session.

## Lorraine: Finding Oneself in the Mist of Bilingual Practices

Being othered due to my Madrileño *acento*/accent in the United States, after immigrating from Spain at the age of 23, was not new for me. As a biracial, Spanish and Black American, woman raised in Spain, I had become familiar with a sense of inadequacy and not being enough. At the age of five, kids in my community made comments that pointed out the color of my skin. Consequently, I was made to believe that I was not enough because my skin color was not sufficiently white for Spaniards. When I moved to the Canary Islands at age 15, I was subjected to hatred and rejection by my peers at school for my *acento Madrileño*. Feeling like an outsider in my own country brought me many times of loneliness. I learned strategies for hiding and blending in before rebelling and finding pride in my *acento, a mucha honra*. I began to accentuate the Madrileño pronunciations of my C, S, and Z sounds as an expression of pride and belonging. I discovered how welcoming it was to live within my accent with its cultural ideologies. It is in my accent where my body and soul are now at home. The journey in search of an identity that will welcome me, therefore, has been the story of my life.

Naively, I believed that becoming a bilingual MFT in the United States was going to be a detour from my identity journey. This bubble quickly burst during my master's training. A sense of loss and confusion ran loose under my skin, flooding my brain with warning signs of inadequacy during my sessions in Spanish. Even though I am a native Spanish speaker, my Madrileño accent and skin color were not apparently white enough in therapy sessions to embody the appropriate professional MFT identity that I was trying to acquire through the program. My Madrileña words were easily available outside of the context of therapy; but in therapy they seemed to have gone into hiding or blended into my English so thoroughly that their color was no longer recognizable. I felt inadequate. I could not display the confidence of my therapeutic identity I gained in English into Spanish. Hence, English started to reign over my sessions in Spanish. I started translating its structure in order to formulate questions, engage clients, and apply techniques. I felt like an imposter, a complete failure.

Then, I once again rebelled against this sense of inadequacy to recover my pride in my Madrileño accent in order to conduct therapy in Spanish. Long and regular conversations with my bilingual cohort mates outside of class helped me reflect upon the differences between our English and Spanish work. This allowed my storytelling Madrileño practices to reemerge and take numerous detours through journeys that build camaraderie through anecdotes and jokes in many colorful Spanish.

## Final Reflections

We deliberately chose to write this chapter as a tapestry of stories woven together by our storytelling traditions. Our decision was twofold. On one hand, we did so as a way to honor and keep alive the oral storytelling traditions of our respective ancestors. Our ancestors entrusted us with the interpretations of their social and cosmological worlds ordered and organized in aesthetic practices (Rivera Cusicanqui 2015), etched in stories, pottery, textiles, and songs. Their legacies teach us that their aesthetic choices are as legitimate as those found in textbooks or research. We intentionally wrote this chapter using the imagery of a tapestry woven with the yarn of our struggles and resistance against monolingualism in the MFT field. It is both a political and aesthetic choice not only to stand up for and preserve the integrity of our linguistic Spanish and Spanglish but also to challenge the current colonial structures, in this case, of the prevalence of MFT training only in English. In this chapter we situate our linguistic aesthetic storytelling practices as legitimate ways to be acknowledged by a scholarly audience rather than having our stories, hence lives, be appropriated, yet again, by an academic platform.

On the other hand, as echoed by our stories, reclaiming the integrity of our linguistic traditions is not only a matter pertinent to writing but crucial to our therapy work in Spanish and Spanglish. The story writing of this chapter also seeks to illustrate the distinct and tangible storytelling aesthetics in our Spanish and Spanglish therapy conversations, as they are filled with accents, imagery, creativity, imagination, symbolism, and humorous detours to address people's suffering. At first, as we mentioned above, working beyond English-configured MFT therapies was not an option for us, as we were so preoccupied with trying to abide by them. Now, we have come to know that our conversations can very well exist in the wonder borderlands of our linguistic identities. This could occur by navigating through choppy waters to arrive at *la frontera* where we no longer need *coyotes del lenguaje* to smuggle past *la migra* their colorful and strong *acentos*.

Even though we came to differentiate and reclaim some of the aesthetic characteristics of our linguistic traditions during our MFT training, this did not take place in the program's academic spaces. We created our community alongside the program and in solidarity with other bilingual therapists. We began to discover how differently we live in English, in Spanish, and in Spanglish borderlands. When our Spanish and Spanglish storytelling practices facilitate heart to heart connections in therapy, we are left feeling breathless *con un nudo en la garganta y con lágrimas en los ojos* – with a knot in our throats and tears in our eyes. Although we hope that our stories have moved you, as they have moved us, we clearly understand that this process is only a peek into a highly complex yet unexplored linguistic understanding on how bilinguality can play out therapeutically.

Our multicultural, social justice training provided us with sophisticated epistemological frameworks to articulate how life is negotiated through complex racial, gender, and social class categories; yet it failed to do the same for bilingualism. It became more evident to us in writing this chapter that our training did not provide a framework by which we could better understand and appreciate the full extent of the complex and sophisticated skills we already possessed and practiced within our borderlands' languages. Most of these knowledge were outside of our own awareness; thus, having intentional spaces to make them visible would have facilitated our migration to other linguistic wonder borderlands of practice. Relying on improvisation and community solidarity, we eagerly anticipate what awaits in our linguistic homelands: not knowing where our intuitions may take us, what accents we might find along the way, or what borders we will be crossing. Yet, we hope that as we continue playing in our linguistic homelands, the MFT field sees and acknowledges that we exist on the other side of its monolingual wall. We entrusted you with our stories with the hope that Anglo borders begin to open and lead to a free flow of languages: by recognizing the legitimacy and standing in solidarity with therapies configured in aesthetic domains other than English.

## References

Anzaldua, G. (1999). *Borderlands: The new mestiza. La frontera* (2nd ed.). San Francisco: Aunt Lute Books.
Foucault, M. (1972). *L'Archéologie du Savoir. L'ordre du discours.* [The archeology of knowledge and the discourse on language (A. Am. Sheridan Smith, Trans.)]. New York: Pantheon Books.
Mohanty, C. T. (2003). *Feminisms without borders: Decolonizing theory, practicing solidarity.* Durham: Duke University Press.
Rivera Cusicanqui, S. (2015). *Sociología de la imagen: Miradas ch'ixi desde la historia andina.* Buenos Aires: Tinta Limón.

# Chapter 4
# *La Questione Della Lingua* Comes to Therapy

**Lodovica Guidarelli**

**Abstract** As a native Italian and Italian-speaking marriage and family therapist practicing in San Diego, clients regularly consult me because of the language I speak. Within this context, I often hear my clients say: "I am another person when I speak Italian." By bringing together my clinical experience, the body of literature of second language acquisition and its interest in the intersection of language acquisition and identity, and the field of narrative therapy and its interest in the discourses of power, decolonization, and identity formation, in this essay I discuss the theoretical implications brought forth by my clients' statement so as to (1) understand and highlight the clinical relevance of those implications and (2) create a space for the emergence of intentional and linguistically responsive therapeutic practices with Italian-speaking clients.

As a native Italian and Italian-speaking marriage and family therapist practicing in San Diego, clients regularly consult me because of the language I speak. Within this context, I often hear my clients say: "I am another person when I speak Italian." In this essay, I explore the theoretical implications brought forth by this statement so as to (1) understand and highlight the clinical relevance of those implications and (2) create a space for the emergence of intentional and linguistically responsive therapeutic practices with Italian-speaking clients.

## From Figure of Speech to Literal Meaning

"I am another person when I speak Italian." I imagine you might have said or heard someone saying something similar, either about Italian or another language. Can you recall who said it, and in what context? Can you remember what they were trying to convey? It is quite a bold statement, and we most often interpret it as a

L. Guidarelli (✉)
Narrative Initiatives San Diego, San Diego, CA, USA



m. polanco et al. (eds.), *Bilingualism, Culture, and Social Justice in Family Therapy*, AFTA SpringerBriefs in Family Therapy,
https://doi.org/10.1007/978-3-030-66036-9_4

hyperbole, a figure of speech that exaggerates an idea for the sake of emphasis. This is how I made sense of it, until I embarked on a new journey to become a therapist. It was in 2012, during my second year of graduate studies in Marriage and Family Therapy at San Diego State University, when I started to entertain the idea that this statement could be taken literally. At that time, I was simultaneously teaching Italian language, literature, and culture at college level, which made me pay attention to how students talk about their experiences of learning Italian; and I was taking a Methods of Research graduate course, which required me to write a research paper on a subject of my choice. I was, thus, living in my own body, a dual linguistic and professional identity, which was as much exciting as it was unsettling since I did not have a language to fully describe and understand it. When I think of that duality, what comes to mind is an image of myself sitting in my car, driving from one university to the other. It seems obvious, now, that I was molting during my commute. It was on the I-8 East freeway, in my PT Cruiser *rossa* (red) that I was shedding the skin of the Italian professor to get ready for the English therapy I was about to offer. I was certainly intrigued by that daily metamorphosis of mine, and the academic assignment for the research class created the perfect space for me to follow my fascination. I, therefore, decided to venture out with two dear classmates of mine in the exploration of what being "another person" meant when speaking a different language in the context of second language acquisition. It wasn't until later, though, when I was presented with the opportunity to work with Italian-speaking clients, who consult with me because of the language I speak, that I returned my attention to this matter anew. This time, it was within a therapeutic context that I heard again and with a different set of ears: "I am another person when I speak Italian." As if coming from a place that was both familiar and mysterious, near and far, different questions started to resurface: what do my clients mean when they say that? What kind of ideas would allow for a literal interpretation of this statement? By engaging these questions, I hope to bring justice to that duality that I still experience in my personal and professional life. It is the duality of a migrant, who is never fully here nor there; whose departures and arrivals are a mix of hope and disappointment, joy and sorrow; who nourishes her body with local produce and foreign recipes and vice versa; and who hears the centuries-old names of her children with the sounds and the promises of the *nuovo mondo*/new world.

## Re-embodying Languages

Some ideas and experiences that support the claim that it is possible to be "another person" when speaking another language come from the field of second language acquisition (SLA). The attention that this field provides to the interaction of two or more languages, and where English acts as the lingua franca, makes SLA a privileged source. As the field has progressively refined and expanded its pedagogical tools to equip instructors to support students interested in acquiring both linguistic proficiency in a foreign language and intercultural competence, research in SLA has engaged in an exploration of the intersection between the acquisition of a second language and the development of identity (Norton 2000, Pavlenko 2005; Block 2007; Kramsch 2009). Among this rich body of literature, the work of Claire Kramsch seems particularly fruitful to my investigation as it explores the subjective experience of learning a foreign language. Her work stands out because, in contrast to most of previous SLA research, Kramsch takes into account the affective component of learning/speaking multiple languages and its effects on identity formation. Rather than confining affectivity into a separate domain of inquiry, one that traditionally would separate body and cognition, Kramsch describes the relationship a multilingual subject entertains with a language as one that "engages their emotions, their bodies, and the most intimate aspects of themselves." (p. 2). She writes:

> As a sign system, language elicits subjective responses in the speakers themselves: emotions, memories, fantasies, projections, identifications. Because it is not only a code but also a meaning-making system, language constructs the historical sedimentations of meanings that we call our 'selves'. (Kramsch 2009, p. 2)

Furthermore, Kramsch notices that not only has language been separated by its own body, but it has also been interpreted as a neutral tool for the formulation of thought and the communication of factual truths and information. In so doing, language has been voided of its own symbolic power, where the term "symbolic" refers "not only to the *representation* of people and objects in the world but to the *construction* of perceptions, attitudes, beliefs, aspirations, values through the use of symbolic forms" (Kramsch 2009, p. 7). In other words, since the symbolic forms of language (its sounds, intonations, linguistic codes, or shapes of the letters) create reality itself, when we access a different language we access a different reality and thus a different identity.

One last concept from Kramsch's work that I find useful in our therapeutic context is the relationship between perception and desire. In her investigation, she defines it as "the need to identify with another reality than the one that surrounds us" and the exploration of the "various possibilities of the self in real or imagined encounters with others." (2009, p. 14). We can state with confidence that when clients come to us seeking support for the predicaments of their lives, they do so because they imagine a different "Other" for themselves being available and achievable and because they are looking to create a different reality from the one that surrounds them. What does that mean for a client that is choosing to seek a different reality and identity in Italian? What imagined realities and identities does their desire to be in therapy in Italian speak about?

As we take into account the body of the language, its symbolic power in its ability to shape different realities and identities, as well as the perception and the desire of an imagined "Other Self," we begin to view the complexity and the richness of the kind of work that is possible when a multilingual client chooses us because of the language that we speak.

## Languages and Power

Kramsch's work is paralleled by a similar shift in the field of marriage and family therapy, in which critical attention has been given to the affective domain of the languages. Although non-structuralist approaches have grounded their philosophical underpinnings on the symbolic power of the language and its ability to create reality, only recently, the work of marcela polanco (2016) has turned a critical eye to the linguistic experiences of multilingual clients. Just as SLA instructors, for years, have focused their attention primarily to the grammatical aspects of languages and their communicative function, similarly, therapists have related to multilanguage clients as if they could simply translate the sought-after information from one language to the other. The assumption was that the result would have been the same. In contrast, through her own journey of translating narrative therapy in her Colombian Spanish, marcela polanco has come to the understanding that narrative therapy was "untranslatable" (2016, p. 69). She needed to engage her flesh-and-body magic realist Colombiana self if she really wanted to access the values and principles of narrative therapy and make them available to her Spanish-speaking clients. In so doing, a new language, new questions, and a new Colombiana narrative therapist identity have become available to her. The creation of a space in which English is no longer privileged allows for the emergence of alternative and subjugated knowledge and identities.

The same is true for our clients and their identities. I would like to argue that when our multilingual clients choose a specific language for their therapeutic conversations, they are privileging a set of knowledge that comes with speaking the language of their choice. It is through the speaking of that chosen language that the experiences, the memories, the sounds, the sensations, and the ideas that shaped that knowledge and that identity become available anew. What kind of knowledge and identity do my Italian-speaking clients have access to when they choose to be in therapy in Italian? Why do they seek that knowledge? What kind of power comes with that knowledge? As we approach our clients' choice of the language with curiosity, we begin to bring justice to the knowledge that comes with those languages, which may otherwise be left outside of the therapeutic space.

## *La Questione Della Lingua*/The Choice of the Language

Who are my Italian-speaking clients? Most of them are multilingual clients, who are fluent in both Italian and English and sometimes in other languages as well. Most of them were born and/or raised in Italy, or that's where they lived a significant part of their life. They associate very personal memories and experiences with each of the languages that they speak. They have lived in the USA for a few or many years. They are connected to their local community, they work in English, they socialize in English, and they may have created bicultural or multicultural families. In most cases, they are not seeking an Italian-speaking therapist because of a linguistic barrier. They are seeking an Italian-speaking therapist because that is what they prefer. When I invite my clients to speak about their linguistic preference, I hear responses that speak to such concerns as: (1) they imagine being better able to talk about their most intimate feelings and sensations, (2) they imagine that an Italian-speaking therapist would be able to understand them better because of the shared culture, and (3) they believe that the Italian-speaking therapist who lives in the USA would be able to act as a cultural broker, especially within the context of relational/family therapy.

My own personal experience with seeking therapy several years ago spoke to similar concerns. My first encounter with psychotherapy happened in the context of my journey as a migrant. I had migrated into the USA a few years before to pursue a Ph.D. in Italian, and I was transitioning into a different stage of adulthood and into my professional identity as a professor of Italian. I remember distinctly the moment in which I decided to seek therapy and the considerations I made. Some of those considerations were about the language. Do I want to be in therapy in Italian or English? What is interesting to notice is that while my logical mind wanted me to choose an Italian-speaking therapist, my body did not. While, on the one hand, I thought that I would have been better able to express myself in Italian, an idea that was accompanied by some sensations of comfort, on the other hand, I was under the impression that I would have come up with some old answers to my old problems. The concept of "old" was coming up as a feeling of heaviness: heavy known ideas, known values, known words, and even known clothes and styles that I did not want to hear or see. I thus came to the conclusion that I preferred an English-speaking therapist because I did not want my therapist to have assumptions about what I valued and because I wanted to "move forward." I was under the impression that a therapeutic relationship with an Italian-speaking therapist would have situated me within the context of the past, instead of the future. Was that true? While as an Italian-speaking narrative therapist I hope not to be the kind of therapist I was portraying in my own imagination, I also recognize that it is not relevant. What is relevant is that I had an idea about how the language I chose would shape my conversations, how I imagined my own change through one language vs. another, and how I associated two identities, sets of knowledge, and physiologies with two different languages. I was in a moment in which I needed to overcome some oppressive ideas that I had learned in Italian, and I imagined being able to succeed by engaging different ideas in a different language. The choice of the language had been shaped by my own story of migration.

There is always a story of migration behind the story of our Italian-speaking clients. I prefer the use of the term migration rather than immigration or emigration because it is never a one-way journey. Just like *le rondini*/swallows with their arrival and departure remind Italians every year that spring and autumn are on their way, my identity as a migrant is defined by a movement between two spaces, in a never-ending cycle of renewal. I remember the day in which I have become a US citizen. The master of the ceremony congratulated every new citizen because on that very day our journey of migration had come to an end. As she was speaking, tears started to stream down my face for the very opposite reason. Through her words, it had just become crystal clear that my journey of migration would have never ended. Just like migration is a necessary act of survival for *le rondini*, that movement of departure and return, both physical and psychological, seems unavoidable for me. It is the very movement through which I re-imagine myself from the perception and desire of the "Other." In my choice of the English-speaking therapist, I was not erasing or trying to forget my Italian identity, I was re-imagining it from the perspective of the US one. The opposite happens as well, that is, when I re-imagine my US identity through the eyes of my Italian one.

Unfortunately, nobody, at the time, approached my very personal *Questione della Lingua* with a curious stance. Would it have been possible to access the hopes, dreams, and aspirations that I was identifying with the choice of the language? While I cannot go back in time, I know that that choice, those feelings, and those reflections have not vanished, and I am only now beginning to see the shining treasure that was hiding underneath them. Who would have ever imagined that a revised *Questione della Lingua*, the seven-century-old debate on which language should be used among the many spoken and written languages of Italy (Hall 2018), would have travelled all the way to San Diego and show up in my therapy room?

## In Search of a Character

In closing her message about *Language Justice*, polanco (2016) invites the readers to embark on a similar journey as hers. She writes:

> In a dreamlike world, I hope that you find your ways to start all over again so as to reimagine new meanings of narrative therapy with new vocabularies, culturally coherent with intentions of language justice. I hope that you find ways, maybe inadvertently, to your own versions of Macondo where you might discover that a new character of your imagination has been waiting for you eagerly with its arms open proceeding to embrace you. (p. 75)

I find the promise of the embrace of a character waiting for me at the end of this journey very captivating. And I don't think it is because I am writing during COVID-19 physical distancing time. I think it is because of the desire I share with the author to bring justice to the richness of each culture, their languages, and the identities that they shape. The allure of this invitation comes also from my love for literature and the arts, especially their transgressive and creative nature, their ability to generate meanings, seek truths, and honor the complexity of our human existence.

My development of linguistically just therapeutic responses is still very young, and the character waiting for me with open arms seem still faceless, just like the mannequins of Giorgio De Chirico and Andrea Savinio's *Scuola Metafisca* (Jewell 2004). Yet, I hope that these pages have offered a preliminary exploration of the possibilities that open up for our clients and us when we consider the body of the language, its symbolic power, the distinct sets of knowledge that come with each language, and their untranslatability. I hope that more practitioners will join me through the perils and the joy of figuring out what bringing language justice to Italian-speaking clients may look like.

## References

Block, D. (2007). *Second language identities*. London, UK: Continuum International Publishing Group.

Hall, R. A. (2018). *The Italian Questione della Lingua: An Interpretative Essay*. Chapel Hill: University of North Carolina Press.

Jewell, K. (2004). *The art of enigma. The De Chirico brothers & the politics of modernism*. University Park: The Pennsylvania State University Press.

Kramsch, C. (2009). *The multilingual subject*. Oxford, UK: Oxford University Press.

Norton, B. (2000). *Identity and language learning. Gender, ethnicity and educational change*. Essex: Pearson Education Limited.

Pavlenko, A. (2005). *Emotions and multilingualism*. Cambridge: Cambridge University Press.

polanco, m. (2016). Language justice: Narrative therapy on the fringes of Colombian magical realism. In *The international journal of narrative therapy and community work* (Vol. 3, pp. 68–73).

# Chapter 5
# Language as Rebellion: Black Folks *Wanna* Speak They Own *Kinda* English in Therapy

**Eureka Vaughn and Candea Mosley**

**Abstract** Most therapy involves dialogical communication; therefore, the language a therapist speaks matters. In an attempt to highlight this complex history of Black American's way of talking, we encourage our reader to have a general knowledge of the role the Trans-Atlantic Slave Trade and Slavery in the United States may have played in contextualizing the Black experience with US English. Due to the oppression of Black people's natural linguistic expression, our intent is to bring awareness to how we as marriage and family therapists (MFTs) can normalize the use of "Black talk" in therapy. We define "Black talk" as a cultural adaptation that rebels against standard English norms and inherently makes one bilingual. As authors, we've chosen to utilize a conversational method to describe our experiences being educated and professional Black women for the sake of offering a glimpse into the challenges we face bringing all of our Blackness into the therapy room.

Black people stand out as we are "never-not" noticed in society. The use of the double negative in that previous sentence is as intentional as the way we speak to one another. For centuries, we have used language as a protest to Western European assimilation and colonization; but before we tackle the complexities of the linguistic history of Blacks in North America, we must first acknowledge the stripping away of the many indigenous African languages. As kidnapped people, West Africans were forced to learn English from their under-educated European captors, which placed them in significant positions of disadvantage (i.e., being considered uneducated due to not speaking "proper English"). Forbidding them from speaking in

E. Vaughn (✉)
ChildNet Youth & Family Services, Long Beach, CA, USA
e-mail: evaughn@childnet.net

C. Mosley
License to Freedom, El Cajon, CA, USA



m. polanco et al. (eds.), *Bilingualism, Culture, and Social Justice in Family Therapy*, AFTA SpringerBriefs in Family Therapy,
https://doi.org/10.1007/978-3-030-66036-9_5

their native tongues (for fear they might organize rebellions), Europeans violently demanded their kidnapped learn an informal, but recognizable way of speaking.

In laying the groundwork for how to describe "Black talk," "Ebonics," or "slang" in this chapter as family therapists, we find it critical to view "Black talk" as a cultural adaptation of the English language so we may position ourselves (Black women raised in both Texas and California) as bilingual. Through time and struggle, Black folks achieved the rights to formal education and the right to learn the "King's English," which in turn afforded more societal advantage. However, if you travel throughout the United States and encounter Black people from varying regions, one gets a clear picture that not only was formalized education of little value to some but that speaking the "Kang's Anglish" (yes, we might sometimes pronounce it as such) was a more overt form of white-washing our West-African heritage and most of us "ain't havin" that, hence the linguistic rebellion.

When rebelling against standard English, our people are oftentimes seen as uneducated and somehow "less-than" and as Black marriage and family therapists (MFTs), we feel a strong sense of responsibility to recognize the importance of this linguistic adaptation for our ancestors, our families, and our clients. Following in this chapter, we position ourselves in reflexive conversation about what it means to talk Black in therapy. For us, there is no way to describe the beautiful rebellion that is "talking Black" without writing a tome. The power we feel knowing we have transformed a "shoved-down-our-throats and thrust upon us," but forbidden, language to make it entirely our own speaks to the rebelling power that is the Black presence in America. We have added to our conversation all of the *flava* from the Motherland, sprinkled with resistance and stirred with a spoon of brilliance, and in doing this it helps us quickly identify who our people are and who they *ain't*.

**Candea:** We spend a lot of time in this academic setting with academic folks and I'm *tryna* create a space for Black therapists to discuss things the way we wanna discuss *'em,* not having to put the "code switch" into white MFT on at all times which can be frustrating because as we're learning these MFT theories there's something blaringly significant: there is little Black representations of people creating this stuff. So I find myself asking how the fuck am I *gonna* explain what I am learning to my mom? How would I help my grandmother understand "externalizing a problem"? Because she'd be like, "Girl if you don't get *outta* my face with that mess." So how do I make our therapy language accessible to folks who only "talk Black" and who don't have access to the MFT standard English? When I'm at home I don't talk like a therapist. If we're inviting people into a room for conversation, we want it to be comfortable as if we are home. But when I come into the therapy room as a therapist, there's a barrier of language created by how I was trained as how I "should" present myself and speak. It feels unnatural.

**Eureka:** So, you're saying there's a totally different language most Black people and Black therapists use when we're in session as opposed to when we're comfortable at home and it's akin to being bilingual. Some call it Ebonics, I call it talking Black, but it's a separate language that has its own nuances and meanings. And this idea of making therapy comfortable makes me wonder, how do we join our Black clients in a way that makes them feel heard and understood? One of the things I've learned is that the main barrier to Black folks seeking services is the lack of therapists understanding them and I reduce that lack of understanding to language.

**Candea:** Yep, I definitely agree. From my lived experience, part of the reason we don't get therapy is because it's hard to go when you're already dealing with so much, adding having to make your therapist understand your language. I had an experience in therapy where I described experiencing coming from a different place and the (non-Black) therapist gave me another word for my description and I was like, that's not what I said and that's not what it means so why are you trying to correct me? And that experience felt offensive and instead of her saying, how can I make my client feel heard and understood, she corrected me in something I'm fluent in, which is my own Black language, *thank you very much*.

**Eureka:** Well that's interesting because it makes me wonder, are Black therapists the only people who fully understand the language of their Black clients? And could that be why Black clients feel most comfortable with Black therapists?

## Respectability of Black Talk (Put Some *Respek* on Our Language)

**Candea:** Well, as black people we've been told that the way we talk is ignorant and wrong, so most therapists I know assume that viewpoint and think that how we're talking is uneducated.

**Eureka:** That's so true. But then you have some Black people who've never even talked "Black" so it goes to show that *them* people don't know us!

**Candea:** But I think non-Black therapists don't even try to get familiar with our language because it's beneath them and unworthy of their time to learn what we're saying.

**Eureka:** I feel you. I'm right there with you. In the Black community, there's this double standard for us because success is tied to education and in order to prove we're educated we tend to speak standard English. We do this "switching" with each other until we get comfortable enough to know if it's cool to let our guard down a lil bit. It's as if we're saying, I'm educated, I got these degrees but I'm *finna* say *dis* how I'm *gon* say it, is that okay? And will you still respect me in the *mornin'*? So much of how we talk gets tied to whether or not we're respectable beings.

**Candea:** I've had people say, "You don't talk like them" and I'm like, what do you mean by them? Are you *talkin'* about my grandpa who was a chauffeur, owned his own business, and knew how to work but couldn't read or write? Who are you talking about? To me, that's the epitome of where we're at with the therapeutic "languaging" piece, especially if we don't speak like them and by "them" I mean White Americans. 'Cause a lot of times people say I "talk white" so then I feel I have to play this game. The way we speak can be a hardship sometimes.

## Talking Black

In an effort to situate this conversation, we use the idea of "talking Black" in direct contrast to "talking White" which reinforces the earlier idea of language as a rebellion. For the purpose of this chapter, we define "talking White" in the same manner that "standard English" is defined in Merriam-Webster's dictionary:

> The English that with respect to spelling, grammar, pronunciation, and vocabulary is substantially uniform though not devoid of regional differences, that is well established by usage in the formal and informal speech and writing of the educated, and that is widely recognized as acceptable wherever English is spoken and understood. (Merriam-Webster 2020, para 1)

We posit that the Black experience is diverse and regions exist where "talking Black" does not.

**Eureka:** When I think about my clients and how my work changes depending on who I'm with, I notice that when I'm with Black clients [primarily children], if I "talk Black" which is more relaxed, less "ings" at the end of words. Fewer "s" on my plurals and more drawn out, elongated vowel sounds, I make an instant connection with them. And what I gather is that although they see I'm Black, I'm still seen as a professional, but when I switch my speech, they see me as one of them.

**Candea:** I work with Middle Eastern folks, and it was important for me to learn some of their language like how to greet them, how to say thank you and use it as a way to connect. I'm an outsider saying, okay, so this means *this* to you. I feel like it's the same way with Black people. Although our language is technically English, we find comfort in connecting through talking Black. And although I'm a therapist, I feel I can even out the linguistic hierarchy by meeting them right where they are.

**Eureka:** So, then I have to ask, do you think minorities are the only people who see language as this important? Are we sensitive to its impact because we know how it feels to be disconnected? Why can't we say the important *thangs* how we *wanna* say *'em*? Can I be with my clients and say *dis* or *dat* because if I were French, I could say *zis* or *zat* and it would be perfectly acceptable. These are the complexities about how Black clients and therapists feel and we *hafta* be conscious of this conundrum existing in the room.

**Candea:** It goes back to the hierarchy of language. We wield knowledge and power when we use the words we use in therapy and it's a privilege. When we're working with minority communities, we wield the power that since we've gone to school, we've gotten our degrees and then we weaponize that power in our language and it's unfair to the clients.

**Eureka:** *Giiiirrrrl, you sho is preachin' now*! I'm thinking about how I just said "conundrum" and I hope I don't say that shit to my clients because it reminds me that language can be oppressive especially if you don't value the language that comes along with formalized education. So, whose language gets prioritized in the therapy room? We *betta* be *allowin'* our clients to speak freely and then comfortable asking for clarity if they say something we don't understand.

## Keeping It Real

As writers, we struggled with identifying the moments that seem ripe for talking Black and with how to present this struggle to other therapists. We agree that Black folks typically feel most comfortable *speakin'* they own kinda English and what that encompasses varies from community to community. We toyed with the idea we call *keepin' it real* which is a Black expression rooted in notions of rejecting political correctness. At the core of talking Black is an essence of "realness" that bonds and connects us to each other. It's a means of survival.

**Eureka:** It's said, "the best way to learn a language is to immerse yourself in the culture and with the people," so I ask, does mainstream US value talking Black as a language? When we met, you and I slipped into a, "hey girrrll," "*mmhmm*" where the intonations and inflections let us know, "I see you. You feel comfortable to me. I understand you." We got alladat from a simple, "Hey girl." So how does this look in therapy? How does, "I see you, I know you, I hear you, I feel you, I've immersed myself with your people, I've learned your language" get communicated?

**Candea:** Well, you have to be invited to the cookout, play dominoes at the table, and beat somebody's ass in spades. I'm from Texas and there's such a thing as speaking *southern*, and it does not equate to being ignorant, but it's funny how "talking Black" somehow does. It's interesting to see this hierarchy in the English language and how we rank at the bottom. Everybody speaks a different *kinda* English.

**Eureka:** When we come in these rooms as therapists and clients, we do feel our language ranks low and there's little room for us to feel safe being ourselves.

**Candea:** As I recently told my MFT professor, in order for me to be respected and taken seriously I have to speak two English languages, White talk and Black talk, and it's a lot of pressure to have to perform at that magnitude all the time. And we put that pressure on ourselves in professional settings in order to survive.

**Eureka:** Something happened at work. I sent a text message to my non-Black boss that I thought I was sending to a Black coworker. The text read: "*phew y'all* something took me out today, it *ain't* the *Rona* (Covid-19/corona virus) but I'm scared than a mug over here. I miss y'all...." When I realized I sent it to my boss, I thought, she's *finna* be like, "Who is this person? Eureka doesn't talk like this," *cause girrrl* all of the colloquialisms *fa sho* came out but when I'm talking to other Black people that's how I feel most comfortable. I was embarrassed and felt exposed but why? You're right, there is a constant pressure to access my academic standard English in the workplace.

**Candea:** Just today I said, "You know what I don't care about this assignment, I'll take the *L* and then I realized I was in class and had to explain that what I meant by *taking the L* was. I was willing to lose my grade point average if I had to. One of the Black guys in the class said, "I love how you just explained *taking the L*."

**Eureka:** We find ourselves interpreting for people if we talk Black and speak in these metaphors and phrases, right? We backtrack and clean it up. Who wants to do that shit all day?

**Candea:** Yeah, we try to legitimize ourselves in that moment because we feel like somehow or another we fell below the curve? Oh shit, let me clean that up so they know I'm this educated woman who's really worked hard to be here. All that *shuckin'* and *jivin'* gets annoying after a while.

**Eureka:** Yes

**Candea:** Honestly if I said I speak two languages: I talk Black and I speak English most people would laugh it off as a joke, but it really isn't.

**Eureka:** And my thinking is, you *gon git alladis* rich Blackness no matter what.

**Candea:** That's definitely a difference because everything I've learned has been through a euro-centric lens. I have friends who, like you, have gone to Black colleges and the thinking is revolutionary. You don't come out of there without no afro. I'm telling you that right now.

**Eureka:** *Rat nah*, as the "country" Black folks would say. I think there's value in both our perspectives. For Black people, proper speech has long been a sign of how well you were raised. If you were raised well, then you were educated and you spoke well. Our use of standard English then dictated our career success or failure, and many of us abandoned talking Black in order to climb a career ladder. I use my Black talk as a form of rebellion, and I wish there were a space for more Black therapists to be comfortable in the therapy room like we are when we're with our families and friends and show up in those ways with our clients.

**Candea:** Yeah, how do we show up with all that blackness in the room? It's a lot and it almost feels unfair cause yes, we have to constantly be two people at one time, at any given time.

**Eureka:** Yep. It's a heavy burden to bear.

## Rebelling with No End

We find there is no conclusion to this ongoing conversation about Language as Rebellion and what it has meant for us as Black therapists. We do know our ancestors used talking Black (the less standardized version of English) as a means of survival. They twisted meanings and words in order to hide plans of escapes and rebellions, and we see that echoed today in Black culture through our music as a means of coded conversation. Our purpose for highlighting this complexity is to offer insight into the Black linguistic experience with the hopes of inviting clinical transparency on the part of a therapist who positions themselves as a non-judgmental ally who seeks to break down the barriers that language can present. We concluded with more questions than answers, yet our goal remains to "do no harm" especially to Black clients who have a rich and difficult linguistic road to navigate. In this war of standard colonization versus *keepin' it real*, our voices prevail and rebel.

## References

Merriam-Webster. (2020). Standard English. In *Merriam-Webster.com dictionary*. Retrieved 16 August, 2020, from https://www.merriam-webster.com/dictionary/Standard%20English

# Chapter 6
# Doing Narrative Therapy in Fenglish

**Navid Zamani and Nadia Zamani**

**Abstract** This chapter will explore the cultural and political terrain that Farsi-speaking therapists navigate when engaging with Farsi-speaking (Iranian Persian) clients utilizing Farsi, English, and *Fenglish*. The authors will situate their own cultural and linguistic locations as Persian Americans and offer practices located in narrative theory. These practices are housed in a poststructuralist translingualism that is interested in the discursive realms of exploring experience as influenced by Western psychological discourse, emerging and ongoing threads of neo colonialism, and broader assumptions of Western counseling on Farsi-speaking therapists. In this chapter, the authors will offer examples and practices that can be considered by therapists with access to Farsi when working with Farsi-speaking clients.

In this chapter, we focus on exploring the practices that have emerged from two Persian American narrative practitioners interested in working with Farsi-speaking clients, necessarily adapting their practice for another language and culture while flexibly maintaining some fidelity to the theoretical and ethical tenets laid out by narrative therapy (White et al. 1990).

We will discuss our journey into these ideas from our particular social locations, provide a brief background on Farsi and narrative therapy, and share the practices that we have been working within therapy contexts. We will be discussing the use of slang Farsi, and specifically Fenglish, to connect to narrative theory throughout this chapter. Our intention is to give credence to the role of slang Farsi and Fenglish as a critical therapeutic language of the Persian diaspora and valuable approach to

We'd like to acknowledge and thank our friends and colleagues for taking time to read and support our work. Thank you Vicki Dickerson, Shirin Eshfagh, Jan Ewing, Kern Haug, Lila Kalaf, Gerald Monk, Niaz Nafisi, and Katie Zamani for your ongoing support and love.

N. Zamani (✉)
San Diego State University, San Diego, CA, USA
e-mail: nzamani@sdsu.edu

N. Zamani
Marriage and Family Therapy, San Diego, CA, USA



m. polanco et al. (eds.), *Bilingualism, Culture, and Social Justice in Family Therapy*, AFTA SpringerBriefs in Family Therapy,
https://doi.org/10.1007/978-3-030-66036-9_6

conducting narrative therapy work. We hope to support other practitioners who may be positioned similarly between Farsi and English to "go for it" by exploring linguistic sensitivities, embracing Fenglish (Farsi English), and resisting discourses of perfection.

## As Persians and Therapists

Our parents migrated to the United States as a result of the Iranian revolution in 1979, eventually settling in Southern California where there is a large Iranian (Persian) diaspora.[1] Besides our parents, our (the authors') family is located in Isfahan, Iran. We visited Iran annually, except for periods when political climates shifted and the risk of being either American or Iranian limited our ability to travel (as is the case at the time of writing this chapter). We learned Farsi first [from our parents] and then English [through the schooling system] while residing in the United States, giving us the experience of moving between two languages, two worlds: two worlds invested in representing the other in particular ways (criminalization, distrust, displacement, colonization, etc.) shaped by a long political history.

We are marriage and family therapists located in San Diego, California, trained in a postmodern program with an emphasis on narrative therapy working with vulnerable communities. We were drawn to narrative ideas and poststructuralist ethics because of its interest in sustaining complexity, storytelling as political, an intentional attention to the linguistic and cultural, and privileging of social justice ethics. We often work with Farsi-speaking clients and we have had to consider forms of practice in Fenglish by necessity.

## Context and Challenges of Narrative Therapy in *Farsi*

The three pillars of the Farsi language include Old Persian, Middle Persian, and Modern Persian, which is what is now considered present-day Farsi (Windfuhr 2011). The Farsi language encompasses the languages of Dari and Tajik.[2] Due to a history of colonization by the French, Germans, and British, there are Indo European words and undertones found in the Farsi language, as well as in the name of the country[3] (Taleghani 2009). For example, *merci* is a word used in Farsi and French that translates to thank you.

[1] We use Persian to refer to a culture distinguished by a history shaped by the Persian empire. Iran is used when referring to the current country whose name and borders are shaped by Western imperialism.

[2] These are dialects of Farsi that are separated due to geopolitical reasons.

[3] Iran is derived from the word, "Aryan," accentuating Iran's complicated relationship with the West (Semaan 1968).

In Farsi, there is a hierarchy consisting of *ketabi* (book/academic) Farsi and *amianeh* (slang) Farsi. Broadly speaking, *ketabi* positions the speaker in an "upper class" and "professional" form of language, while *amianeh* associates the user as uneducated and/or of a lower socioeconomic level. Each region and city has its own form of *amianeh*, often with attached stereotypes. Fenglish has become a derivative of *amianeh* Farsi used by the Iranian diaspora in English-speaking countries. The use of Fenglish is distinguished by a mixture of Farsi and English words to construct sentences, as access to particular words or culturally loaded terms become intentionally selected, and the use of English letters to transliterate Farsi words.

## *Access to* Ketabi, Amianeh, *and* Fenglish

Speaking *ketabi* typically requires access to education in a formal Iranian institution, where students are engaging with literature and knowledge located firmly within *Farsi*. For Iranian diaspora, without formal pedagogy, we are only inculcated with *amianeh* through our family. Within *amianeh*, there are still particular scripts that indicate politeness, respect, and hospitality which are culturally learned. In spaces dominated by English and where opportunities to speak and be educated in *Farsi* are marginalized, *Fenglish* can serve as an important bridge between native *Farsi* speakers and those in the Persian diaspora who don't have access to *ketabi* Farsi.

We have noticed in our use of *Fenglish* that this particular language can open up many relational doors with Persians we serve, while also inviting a sense of uncertainty of our "professionalism" and cultural identities. While this uncertainty can be a barrier to practitioners using *Fenglish* with clients, we will discuss how to lean into these uncertainties by being transparent with clients, remaining curious about different meanings and words, privileging Farsi expressions, and normalizing our uncertainties that may come up.

## Practices for Conducting Narrative Therapy with Fenglish

### *Acknowledging Iran's History*

It is important to acknowledge the histories of oppression that constitute Iranian history. We prioritize culturally reflexive practices where our social locations and histories are named so that these power structures are held accountable in the counseling room (Monk et al. 2020). For instance, when I (Navid) work with Afghan Farsi-speaking clients, I acknowledge the longstanding fraught history between Iranians and Afghans. The onus of responsibility lies on the clinician to be transparent about the potential of these power structures, as these histories can hold lots of pain with little to no opportunity to confront and speak with the "other." Even in the United States, we are forced to confront geopolitical histories from the Middle East that extend before and beyond us, shaped by imperialism, classism, and North/South global relations (Bouteldja 2016).

### *The Challenge of English*

English is a language of trade and conquest, spread with capitalism and harboring British values located in commerce like efficiency, productivity (being "to the point"), and muted expressions of emotion (Diversi and Moreira 2016; polanco 2016a). Farsi is described as "flowery," "emotional," or "dramatic."

Offering clients the ability to speak and share stories in Farsi gives access to a colorful world sometimes not accessible to English-only speakers. A Fenglish-speaking therapist's acute attention to privileging expressions in Farsi and locating them firmly within meaning-making systems can allow for a richer expression of lived experiences and enable a decolonial spirit in the work.

### *Negotiating Social Justice*

Positioning with social justice praxis in our work as narrative therapists requires broader considerations of power and influence when working with Iranian immigrants and the Persian diaspora. Farsi and other languages are forced to respond to the emergence of particular social justice issues located in English (i.e., Western feminism). An application of contemporary Western social justice issues can inadvertently replicate Western imperialism disguised as social justice (e.g., vaccinations by NGOs in Pakistan as a covert operation to gather DNA to locate Osama bin Laden). Instead, we can harness stories of resistance, progressiveness, inclusivity, and community action from Persian history to support meaningful constructions of identity for Persians.

## Working with Narrative Ideas in *Farsi*

Narrative therapy, as a framework, explicitly infused broader political and sociological knowledge sourced in postmodernism, poststructuralism, and critical feminist theory into therapy. In this exploration, we have discovered that Farsi holds many useful intersections with narrative ethics and principles even while its specific application takes on a distinct form.

## *Expanding Notions of Identity Within Family*

Farsi privileges family structure and relationships. Families are significant in how they shape relationships, and there are often distinct hierarchies and roles located by age, gender, and professional experience. Performances of identity are often shaped by broader familial politics, and the interpretations of identity (e.g., reputation) are shaped by actions of family members. For example, Persian children who achieve high levels of education reflect their success onto their entire family, and tragically, the converse is also true.

## *Negotiating Language*

Transparency about our own language abilities is an important point of connection. Humbly describing our own histories with Persian culture and naming our Farsi abilities and hopes for a relationship can create a collaborative effort. "Wondering about words" with clients can create a beautiful "portrait of culture," where the negotiations of language and culture become visible and active (m. polanco, personal communication, 2020).

The chasm between native Persian Farsi speakers and Persian American Fenglish speakers presents an opportunity. We have identified three methods in which we negotiate language and "come to know" about words with our clients, as follows.

**Asking Our Client** Narrative therapists have a common practice to ask clients for permission to inquire about common practices of their lives (Zimmerman and Dickerson 1996), which emulates customs of Iranian hospitality. Our inquiry for a definition is nestled within narrative therapy's deconstructive questions to understand distinctions with other words and, in doing so, shaping the storying of experiences. If our client has access to English or another language, this deconstruction is invited across languages. For instance, a client who shared about considering divorce was invited [by Navid] to reflect on the implications of the word *taalagh*, or divorce, in its respective language/culture. The "personal" choice to divorce was more clearly situated within the political parameters of two languages. The bundles of discourses and meanings that are associated with this word are explored and deconstructed.

**Web-Based Translation Services** This practice is required when the therapist recognizes that using Fenglish or asking the client can interrupt a flow in the dialogue. The practice of using web-based translation services is used with permission from our clients. It typically requires a discussion prior and an explicit agreement about how a computer or smartphone will be utilized in session, with explicit considerations of confidentiality. When using a smartphone with Google Translate™, we download the language dictionary, turn off tracking and history, and disconnect from Wi-Fi/mobile networks. Using translation services en vivo creates a collaborative effort of "figuring it out," as well as naming and noticing that there is often *not* a direct translation.

**Exploring Words Outside of Therapy** A tension in asking a client to define words is that the therapists' efforts may inadvertently privilege the translation process over the storytelling process. For clients who are recounting stories with momentum, it can be disruptive to pause and ask for a word. In these instances, we have our own shorthand note taking by writing words down in Fenglish so that we may ask the client later or ask our own family members who speak Farsi. When asking family members, it's important to eventually circle back to the client to find an experience near definition located within the client's linguistic world. This process has been a beautiful point of connection, personally, with our own family, and an entry point into many family stories that were previously buried. This reflects the narrative therapy theoretical notions of linking lives and outsider witness practice, a narrative therapy practice where intersections of stories between clients and client/therapist are noticed and privileged (Carlson 2020).

## *Externalization*

Externalization is a practice where the use of verbs and adjectives to describe oneself is shifted to a noun form. The effort is to separate the problem from the person and create a linguistic space to consider the relationship one has with the identified problem (White 2007). Externalization tends to function well in Farsi. Farsi tends to locate experiences in parts of the body, such as organs. The Cartesian duality of mind/body located in English is not as prominent. Rather, the emphasis is often on the *rooh* (spirit) which means the fullness of the mind/body and spirit of the human experience. Within these descriptions of experience are cultural values. For instance, the word *del* encompasses both the "heart" and the "stomach" depending on context.

## *Use of Metaphor and Storytelling*

The use of metaphor is a critical linguistic tool ingrained into Farsi and Persian culture and a practice privileged in narrative therapy. Metaphor, similar to externalization, offers a linguistic and visual vehicle in which to explore concepts, processes, and interpretations of the world that resists the person being the problem.

It is common in *mehmoonis* (family gatherings/parties) that dinner is followed by recitations of poetry by various attendees, typically starting with elders. Our own interest in the use of metaphor as narrative therapy practitioners has been shaped by this history. Using the metaphors of human organs as active participants in the shaping of emotion and/or cultural stories that shape discursive terrains can be harnessed to explore landscapes of action, meaning, identity, and physiology while identifying preferences.[4] For instance, *asaub am khoord shod* translates to "my nerves were shattered" (I became angry); *del am tang shod* translates to my "heart became tight" (I miss [somebody]).

A benefit of Persian stories is an emphasis on the storytelling and the process of the characters. Unlike dominant storytelling culture in the United States, there is often not a clear protagonist or antagonist, no clear resolution or "happy ending," nor is there a clearly laid out moral to be easily digested. Persian storytelling allows for therapeutic conversations that honor the complexity and multiplicity of stories and identities and an invitation for clients to apply a similar ethic in constructing and understanding their own lives (Peseschkian 1986).

## Conclusion

Conducting Farsi in therapy sessions with a narrative therapy and postmodern approach creates many challenges and opportunities. Embracing mistakes in the language allows for opportunities of connection and deconstruction. As bilingual clinicians, we are privileged to bear witness to the lives of first-generation Iranians and to their "portraits of culture." The Farsi language allows access to this portrait in ways English cannot; it embodies the experience of the *rooh*. Our hopes are for bilingual (or Farsi-speaking) clinicians to lean into linguistic sensitivities, embrace Fenglish, explore meanings of words, and resist discourses of "perfection" in language.

## References


Bouteldja, H. (2016). *Whites, Jews and us*. South Pasadena: Semiotext (e).

Carlson, T. S. (2020). Who is the outsider in insider and outsider witnessing practices? *Journal of Narrative Family Therapy*. IWP Special Release. 5 15.

Diversi, M., & Moreira, C. (2016). *Betweener talk: Decolonizing knowledge production, pedagogy, and praxis*. Routledge, Walnut Creek, CA.

Monk, G., Winslade, J., Sinclair, S., & Polanco, M. (2020). *Intercultural counseling: Bridging the us and them divide*. Cognella.

Moreira, C., & Diversi, M. (2012). Betweeners speak up: Challenging knowledge production through collaborative writing and visceral knowledge in decolonizing times. *International Review of Qualitative Research, 5*(4), 399–406.

Peseschkian, N. (1986). *Oriental stories as tools in psychotherapy: The merchant and the parrot*. Springer-Verlag: Berlin.


[4] We encourage you to read White's (2007) *Maps of Narrative Practice* for more information about statement of position maps, scaffolding practices, and identifying preferences within these landscapes of experience.

polanco, m. (2016a). Language justice: Narrative therapy on the fringes of Colombian magical realism. *International Journal of Narrative Therapy & Community Work, 3*, 68.
Semaan, K. I. (1968). *Linguistics in the middle ages: Phonetic studies in early Islam*. Leiden: Brill Archive.
Taleghani, A. H. (2009). Persian linguistics in the twentieth century. *Iranian Studies, 42*(2), 275–284.
White, M. K. (2007). *Maps of narrative practice*. WW Norton & Company.
White, M., White, M. K., Wijaya, M., & Epston, D. (1990). *Narrative means to therapeutic ends*. New York: London.
Windfuhr, G. L. (2011). *Persian grammar: History and state of its study* (Vol. 12). Stuttgart: Walter de Gruyter.
Zimmerman, J. L., & Dickerson, V. C. (1996). *If problems talked: Narrative therapy in action*. New York: Guilford Press.

# Chapter 7
# Therapeutic Latinx Story-Sharing or Chismorreo

**Carlos A. Ramos, Jimena Castro, and Joseph Alvaro Guerrero Velez**

**Abstract** Through the lens of de Cervantes's classic Spanish novel, *Don Quijote de la Mancha*, we discuss the nature of language and reality and the idea of therapeutic story-sharing or *chismorreo* (gossiping). Within the Latinx community, the oral practice of *chismear* or *chismorrear* is a common communicational practice that involves imagination, fascination, and novelty (Tanaka, *Fermentum. Revista Venezolana de Sociología y Antropología 17*:646–672, 2007). In this chapter, we explore how Spanish-speaking marriage and family therapy (MFT) supervisors and therapists, at Our Lady of the Lake University, San Antonio, embrace their novelistic imagination to explore clients' resourceful identities, peripheral stories, and undefined journeys.

In this chapter, we[1] focus on our linguistic practices as bilingual (Spanish/English) family therapists working in academic and clinical settings. Within these contexts, we have been challenged with the question of figuring out how to switch codes between English and Spanish. We (Carlos and Jimena) received our marriage and family therapy (MFT) training in English, and we are now teaching, supervising, and doing clinical work in both English and Spanish at Our Lady of the Lake University (OLLU), San Antonio. Alvaro is currently finishing his MFT training and Psychological Services for Spanish Speaking Populations certificate at OLLU and has been seeing clients in both English and Spanish at our university-sponsored community clinic. In the process of doing this, we have encountered issues of

[1] We, Carlos, Jimena, and Alvaro, embrace the term Latinx to refer to our linguistic and cultural commonalities while also embracing our cultural idiosyncrasies. Born in Venezuela to Cuban parents, Carlos emigrated to Miami as a toddler. Jimena is from Cali, Colombia, and she has been living in the USA for over 10 years. Alvaro was born in Mexico and emigrated to Texas as a child.

C. A. Ramos (✉) · J. Castro
Our Lady of the Lake University, San Antonio, TX, USA
e-mail: caramos@ollusa.edu

J. A. G. Velez
Nova Southeastern University, Fort Lauderdale, FL, USA



m. polanco et al. (eds.), *Bilingualism, Culture, and Social Justice in Family Therapy*, AFTA SpringerBriefs in Family Therapy,
https://doi.org/10.1007/978-3-030-66036-9_7

untranslatability, as polanco (2016) suggested: the words and meanings we construct and perform in "one language often becomes inaccessible or untranslatable to be performed in the other" (p. 69). Thus, rather than translating therapeutic ideas and questions from one language to the other, we have engaged our imaginations as polanco invited. For this, we have drawn ideas from de Cervantes's classic Spanish novel, *Don Quijote de la Mancha* (2004). We have also allowed the flair of the Latinx social practice of *chismorrear, chismosear, or chusmear* (i.e., gossiping)[2] to flow through our conversations and therapeutic practices.

## Bakhtin, Don Quijote, and the Art of Story-Sharing

Bakhtin (1981) suggested that "Language—like the living concrete environment in which the consciousness of the verbal artist lives—is never unitary" (p. 288). He casted light on the multi-voicedness of dialogical engagement, and he considered the novel as the quintessential genre in which this polyphony can take place. According to Villanueva (in de Cervantes 2015), the classic novel *Don Quijote de la Mancha* is an example of Bakhtin's *dialogism*, or "dialogue between languages" (p. xvi). In Don Quijote, de Cervantes (2004, 2015) weaves in multiple narrator voices, dialogues between the different characters, between the author and his creation, and various idiosyncrasies, slangs, and expressions informed by different senses. The pattern of interaction among the characters revolved around the exchange of stories and experiences, regardless of "reality," objectivity, truthfulness, and/or sanity.

This contested idea of sanity or reality is mainly depicted in Cervantes's main character, Don Quijote, who, as an expert in the antiquated practice of chivalry, "created a self-image from books…of heroic deeds of medieval knights" (Slade 2004, p. 55). Under this pretense, Quijote embarked on an elusive journey to combat evil or as he claimed, "to extirpate such a wicked race from the face of the [E]arth" (de Cervantes 2004, p. 55). Along with befriending neighborhood countryman Sancho Panza, Don Quijote interacted with a variety of other characters with rich and detailed stories during his heroic quest. Despite that others questioned Quijote's reality, they also engaged in the art of vividly telling their stories. One of them, Cardenio, whom the local goatherd considered a "lunatic," shared his story of misfortune with Don Quijote. Cardenio had taken refuge in the Sierra Morena, a remote and rural area in the mountains, after having discovered that he was betrayed by his compadre Don Fernando, who exploited his position of wealth and power to enamor Cardenio's one true love, Luscinda. "Listen[ing] with vast attention" (de Cervantes 2004 p. 182), Don Quijote "promised, in behalf of himself and the company, to

[2] The words *chismorrear, chismear*, or *chusmear* will be used interchangeably throughout this chapter. These words are used in different Latin American countries to refer to the linguistic and sociocultural practice of telling *chismes*, that is, of sharing intimate stories about others who are not present (Tanaka 2007). We are using the word gossiping as the closest translation in English; however, we acknowledge that the felt sense of the *chismear* cannot be captured in translation.

avoid all manner of interruptions" (p. 183). As a result of their plurilinguistic engagement, the characters' identities and aspirations transformed as they shared their stories and realities yet to never be the same.

## Language(s) and the Construction of Reality

Social constructionists emphasize the role of language in the construction of reality (Gergen 2015). The language we speak shapes our perception, the ways we describe experiences or construe events (Boroditsky 2011). For instance, "bilinguals change how they see the world depending on which language they are speaking" (p. 65). This is evident in the therapeutic context, in which bilingual and multilingual clients may bring forward different selves when they switch languages (Rolland et al. 2017).

As bilingual (English/Spanish and Spanglish) family therapists, we have been ruminating with questions related to the unique qualities that our journey across languages brings to the conversations with our clients. We have been wondering what happens in our traveling back and forth "in the space in between . . . [the] distinct and particular visions of life" (polanco 2016, p. 69) that our languages bring and in the plurilinguistic dialogues in which we engage. In this quest, we and our students have noticed that our ways of engaging in therapy have a unique taste depending on the language we speak; our story-sharing in Spanish has a different pace, emotionality, logic, flow, and so on. We have also recognized that our conversations are not always straightforward or linear. Thus, to help us describe our dialogical practices, we became curious about what the practice of *chismorreo* entailed.

## Latinx Therapeutic *Chismorreo*

Some authors (e.g., Fasano et al. 2009; Tanaka 2007) have pointed to the sociocultural, therapeutic, and identity constitutive functions of the Latinx practice of *chismorreo*, *chusmear*, and *chismear* (i.e., gossiping).[3] Tanaka (2007) considered it as a social and dialogical practice, in which the participants tell, create, and reconstruct the information that is passed on. The practice of *chismorreo* usually happens in small groups where participants know and trust each other. They gossip about people who are not present, and the stories they tell transform as they are being told (Tanaka 2007, p. 650). The accuracy or the truthfulness of the stories is irrelevant. In the process of sharing them, they become real.

---

[3] In a review of the literature, Tanaka (2007) noted that the practice of gossiping has been studied in different social contexts throughout history. Some studies focused on highlighting negative and serious consequences of the practice (e.g., moral sanction and public humiliation), whereas others have pointed toward its positive aspects (e.g., promoting friendship and facilitating group cohesion, among others).

Similar to the art of story-sharing in Don Quijote, with its sensory details and plurilinguistic richness, Latinx *chismorreo* also involves imagination, fascination, and novelty. In addition to its social function, the practice of *chismorrear* has also been deemed therapeutic. It opens the dialogical space for the participants to connect with each other and to embrace the complexities of human's thoughts and emotions (Tanaka 2007). This communicational practice allows the participants to understand themselves within the context of a community (Fasano et al. 2009). Explaining the practice through Bakhtin's ideas, Fasano et al. (2009) suggested that through the *chusmeo*, the participants construct the other in reference to who they are and vice versa. They engage in a relational discursive practice, which "doubleness" allows them to *ser de acá* y *ser diferente* (to be from here and to be different) (p. 75).

## Our Story-Sharing

> The world is nothing if not stories, stories we tell ourselves to live.
> (Stavans 2018, p. 55)

Let us introduce you to *unos chismes*, or a few stories, about our clinical experiences. We hope to bring the spirit of Don Quixote, Sancho Panza, and a few other characters in Cervantes's novel, whose plurilinguistic engagement allowed them to experience themselves differently (to be transformed), as they crossed back and forth between their realities. Like the characters in Don Quixote, our Spanish-speaking clients vividly and passionately share their (most often elaborate and emotional) stories. They invite us into their world through narratives about themselves and/or others or, as we have described, therapeutic *chismorreo*. Through these stories, we get a better understanding of our clients' dreams, hopes, struggles, experiences, relationships, worldviews, purpose, and so on.

While our clients share their stories, we tend to adopt a Don Quixote stance, in which we listen with "vast attention" (de Cervantes 2004, p. 182). We would describe, however, our listening posture as having a novelistic intention. We listen "with an openness to hearing the clients' stories more than listening for symptoms or to develop insight" (Hibel and Polanco 2010, pp. 51–52) while participating with our clients in a plurilinguistic story-sharing.

## *Chismeando con Lina*[4]

A woman (Lina), who lost her husband a while ago, came to our clinic. Lina mentioned that she and her adult children have been coping with their pain by supporting each other. Family was very important to them. While explaining how all the fingers in a hand relate to each other, she described her family. We acknowledged and validated her family's ability to work together. Then, we became curious about what had brought her to our clinic. Lina had been really sick and close to dying. While in the hospital, she had lost consciousness and was in what she understood the process of dying. She found herself in darkness but then saw a light and a tunnel. Her husband was there extending his hand. He seemed to be at peace. Lina felt compelled to take his hand and follow him, but suddenly, she remembered her children. As soon as this happened, she could not see her husband anymore and was awakened (came back to life). Since then, she has been feeling "culpable" (guilty). She felt guilty for coming back to life and not following him, and she also felt guilty about her guilt because she should have not desired this.

Midway through the session, we decided to conduct a reflecting team (Andersen 1987). In a reflecting team, the team members usually comment on what they have learned from the client and share their curiosities about the situation, while the clients listen to the conversation. Although reflecting teams are very common in MFT training settings, therapists have approached them in various ways depending on their intentionality and therapeutic assumptions. In our experimenting with them, we have noticed that our ways of reflecting have changed because of our work with Spanish-speaking clients. We embrace our clients as if we were in a family gathering. Some of us might sit on the floor, if there are not enough spaces for all of us. We might be quite loud and *dicharacheros* (i.e., chatty) or serious and solemn, depending on the situation. There are no strict rules about how this dialogue needs to unfold; however, the team members usually reflect on what they have heard from the client and how the clients' stories have touched them (us). We do this while sharing our own personal and professional stories. Jimena, for instance, shared a story of her father whose right thumb had been amputated when he was diagnosed with melanoma 10 years ago. From writing to grabbing things, everything was a struggle for him, and it was also painful. He suffered from phantom limb pain. He got mad and sad; yet somehow, he kept going while re-learning how to work with his four-fingered hand.

Similar to what happens in the practice of chismorreo, we related to Lina's stories from our own vantage point. This positioning allowed us to be with her and to be ourselves, to cross back and forth between our realities. As Fasano et al. (2009) suggested, *ser de acá y ser diferente* (to be from here and to be different) (p. 75).

---

[4]The conversation with Lina was conducted in Spanish. The team members who participated during the initial conversation included the co-therapists (Alvaro and Erric), the supervisor behind the mirror (Jimena), and four other therapists in training (i.e., Celeste, Ann, Areli, and Valerie). During the follow-up session, Carlos was the supervisor behind the mirror.

Immersed in our plurilinguistic engagement with Lina, we acknowledged the complexity of her situation and reflected on her family's values and strengths. We also sprinkled some novel elements and shared our doubts about her interpretation of what her husband may have wanted to communicate in her dream by extending his hand. As Fasano et al. (2009) noted, for *chisme* to be possible there needs to be an "undefined" territory (p. 78). It is in this undefined territory where new stories can be born. We acknowledged that it made sense that she had thought that her husband wanted her to follow him, given how close they were, and we also wondered out loud if perhaps he wanted to communicate something else. Given that he seemed peaceful in her dream, we suggested that perhaps he wanted to tell her he was fine, so she could continue her life. Our client told us that she had not thought about it in that way but that it was certainly a possibility because her husband cared for her and her family. During the follow-up session, Lina appeared to be relaxed. Her concern about her dream and decision to remain in this world was no longer a concern.

## *Chismeando con Lazara and Juan*[5]

This *chisme* is about two Mexican Spanish-speaking parents (Juan and Lazara) who had a story to share. They wanted their son (Armando) to quit smoking marijuana because of its hallucinatory effects. Armando was never physically present in any of the sessions, but his story (*chisme*) was salient despite his absence. In the initial session, they described a variety of pathological ways that marijuana provoked insanity in their son, which included hallucinations, paranoia, and distancing himself from friends. Although most of the descriptions of Armando had negative connotations, we listened with vast attention and curiosity.

Buried within these pathological descriptions, the therapists discovered Armando's dream of becoming a farmer and being able to economically provide for his parents in the future. As the focus shifted to Armando's aspirations, the topic of marijuana became less of a concern. Juan and Lazara then felt a sense of comfort with the therapists and shared their personal *chismes*. Juan mentioned that he had always worked hard and spent 12–14 hours on his farm developing his agriculture. Lazara's story revolved around religion and her devotion to the Catholic church, as well as her role as a mother, having raised two magnificent children.

We wondered about Juan's strengths, his work ethic, in relation to Armando's aspirations to become a farmer and his dedication to provide for his parents. Juan mentioned that Armando used to help out at the farm. However, because of his marijuana use and abnormal behaviors, Juan and Lazara thought it was safer for Armando to stay home. Although we understood their concern, we asked Juan if he would be willing to try an experiment. The experiment was to choose any day of the week in

[5] In this chisme, Alvaro was one of the therapists, and Carlos was the supervisor observing behind the one-way mirror. All conversations were in Spanish.

which Juan felt safe and comfortable inviting Armando to the farm to help with the labor. The second part of this experiment, which was a bit more unusual, was to remain open and receptive to any conversations or topics that could come up. Essentially, we were asking Juan to curiously immerse himself in Armando's reality with the intention of allowing his son to tell his story, regardless of the "truthfulness" or "sanity" of it. Some would say that we suggested a Don Quijote and Sancho Panza relationship, in which two different realities (or understandings of the world) were able to converge.

We provided a similar suggestion to Lazara. Curious about the family's devotion to Catholicism, we wondered if they spoke about God or prayed at home. Lazara said that she wanted to dedicate more time to praying for Armando, so we suggested if she would be willing to pray with him about any concern, regardless of the concern. A few weeks after these suggestions, Juan and Lazara described a variety of changes. Juan mentioned that he invited Armando to the farm and both had worked most of the week. Juan provided a specific example of how he was able to immerse himself in Armando's reality. While working, Armando mentioned that he felt uncomfortable because there were people watching and criticizing him. Rather than trying to persuade Armando otherwise, Juan listened and agreed with Armando that others were watching and criticizing but because they were envious of his work ethic. Juan mentioned that Armando agreed and continued to work.

Lazara said she was able to spend more time with Armando. They started to randomly pray throughout the day and continued to go to church on Sundays. In our last session, Lazara mentioned that a priest randomly approached them and recommended that they should believe their son's unique experiences because the devil does exist. The priest had now become a part of this plurilinguistic engagement. At that moment, Lazara mentioned that she became more understanding and accepting of Armando's experiences, and what they thought was insanity was a reality they were initially unable to understand.

## Closing Comments

When we engage with our clients in some sort of therapeutic *chismorreo*, we are not concerned with the trueness or sanity of their stories but with creating a dialogical space for our voices to create together. Latinx MFTs could be inspired to embrace their clients' *chismes* and explore with them undefined territories. By means of their novelistic imagination, therapists and clients could share *chismes*, stories, metaphors, ideas, and therapeutic suggestions.

## References

Andersen, T. (1987). The reflecting team: Dialogue and meta-dialogue in clinical work. *Family Process, 26*, 415–428.

Bakhtin, M. M. (1981). *The dialogic imagination. Four essays*. Austin: The University of Texas Press.

Boroditsky, L. (2011). How language shapes thought. *Scientific American, 304*, 62–65.

de Cervantes, M. (2004). In C. Slade (Ed.), *Don Quixote. (T. Smollet, Trans.)*. New York: Barnes and Noble Classics Series.

de Cervantes, M. (Edición Conmemorativa). (2015). Prólogo a la segunda edición del IV Centenario. Don Quijote de la Mancha (pp. xiii–xxxii). New York: Random House Grupo Editorial.

Fasano, P., Ruiu, A., Giménez, J. M., Ramírez, A., Aymá, A., & Savulsky, N. (2009). El sentido del chisme en una comunidad de pobres urbanos. Ciencia, Docencia y Tecnología, 39, (Año XX), 49–85.

Gergen, K. J. (2015). *An invitation to social construction* (3rd ed.). New York: Sage Publishing.

Hibel, J., & Polanco, M. (2010). Tuning the ear: Listening in narrative therapy. *Journal of Systemic Therapies, 29*(1), 51–66. https://doi.org/10.1521/jsyt.2010.29.1.51

polanco, m. (2016). Language justice: Narrative therapy on the fringes of Colombian magical realism. *The International Journal of Narrative Therapy and Community Work, 3*, 68–76.

Rolland, L., Dewaele, J. M., & Costa, B. (2017). Multilingualism and psychotherapy: Exploring multilingual clients' experiences of language practices in psychotherapy. *International Journal of Multilingualism, 14*(1), 69–85.

Stavans, I. (2018). *Don Quixote of La Mancha*. University Park: The Pennsylvania State University Press.

Tanaka, C. (2007). El chisme como fenómeno social: un campo-tema desde la perspectiva construccionista. *Fermentum. Revista Venezolana de Sociología y Antropología, 17*(50), 646–672.

# Chapter 8
# A Meeting of Languages: English-Based Trauma and Spanish Language Variations

**Nidya Ramirez Ibarra**

**Abstract** This chapter centers the author's identity as a bilingual psychotherapist serving Spanish-speaking Latinx clients who have survived intimate partner violence or sexual assault. This chapter challenges the idea that cultural competency with Latinx Spanish speakers is accomplished by providing services based on translation and interpretation from English to Spanish. Significant aspects of a client's Spanish language and sociopolitical and cultural experiences can be neglected in the process of translating and interpreting. This will be accomplished by considering a therapeutic relationship with bilingualism, specifically the Spanish language. The author discusses practices and thought processes that are incorporated into therapeutic work to shift away from traditional translation and interpretation practices. The author will share reflections and observations that have impacted efforts to create a psychotherapy process, particularly addressing experiences of trauma in relationship to Spanish language variations and sociopolitical and cultural realities.

Ideas and practices that I embody as a bilingual psychotherapist are constantly evolving. Recently I have been confronting and struggling with the reality that English-based knowledge dominates my experiences within community, education, and psychotherapy. Implicit and explicit focus on translation and interpretation in community and educational settings reinforces and normalizes English-based knowledge as a neutral and unquestionable foundation. This realization evolved out of therapeutic conversations with my Spanish-speaking Latinx clients. We meet at a domestic violence and sexual assault organization that centers dominant trauma discourses and transfers neurobiology paradigms from the English to Spanish language. These traditional structures of translating and interpreting revealed in them a need to connect Spanish Latinx psychotherapy services to the sociopolitical, cultural, and collective experiences of the community being served. I am actively and constantly devising strategies and questions that can assist in prioritizing Spanish

N. R. Ibarra (✉)
San Diego, CA, USA



m. polanco et al. (eds.), *Bilingualism, Culture, and Social Justice in Family Therapy*, AFTA SpringerBriefs in Family Therapy,
https://doi.org/10.1007/978-3-030-66036-9_8

language variations and Latinx immigrant experiences in psychotherapy which stand outside of dominant English-based trauma narratives.

## Spanish Language and Justice for the Latinx Community

I transitioned into working with an exclusively Spanish-speaking client caseload at a local trauma-focused organization after completing my education and training entirely in English as a postmodern psychotherapist. At the local organization, many hours of staff training are dedicated to becoming an expert on experiences of trauma from a neurobiology and post-traumatic stress disorder perspective. An expectation exists for these ideas to be instilled into the psychotherapists' lens. The premise is that neurobiology knowledge related to trauma holds proven truths about the suffering of all clients regardless of their language or cultures. Bessel van Der Kolk, Daniel Siegel, and Peter Levine are lauded in the organization as the founders and leaders of neurobiology and experiences of trauma; yet they are White men producing knowledge in the English language. In *The Body Keeps the Score: Brain, Mind, and Body in the Healing of Trauma*, van Der Kolk (2014) initiates the book by summarizing that

> ...overwhelming experiences affect our innermost sensations and our relationship to our physical reality-the core of who we are...trauma is not just an event that took place sometime in the past; it is also an imprint left by that experience on mind, brain, and body. This imprint has ongoing consequences for how the human organism manages to survive in the present. (Van der Kolk 2014, p. 21).

He then continues by presenting client cases and research conclusions that lack connections to the role of language, socioeconomic status, race, ethnicity, or sexual orientation in experiences of trauma. Instead, throughout van Der Kolk's links between trauma, the brain, and the body, there are essentialist notions such that the stories of trauma represent and exemplify a collective human experience of suffering. Essentialism is defined as "...fundamental attributes that are conceived as internal, persistent, and generally separate from the ongoing experience of interaction with the daily socio-political contexts of one's life (Bohan 1993, p. 7)." Lived and embodied experiences of trauma though are tied to the particularities of navigating life in specific languages and cultures (White and Epston 1990).

The story of Gloria, a past client (whose name and details I modified), represents the convergence of trauma and systemic injustices in the lives and bodies of many Spanish-speaking clients. Gloria revealed living with hypervigilance and anxiety in her body as she attempted to maintain a job that allowed her to support her family despite her limited English and undocumented status. She explained that for many months she endured rape and sexual assault from a manager and did not immediately report the sexual assault to the police. The fear of "ICE" (Immigration and Customs Enforcement) possibly becoming involved and separating her family was emotionally and physically daunting. Gloria revealed that feelings of desperation led her to report the sexual abuse to the police in her limited English. It is common for Spanish-speaking clients I work with to persistently situate systematic injustices in the experiences and effects of intimate partner violence or sexual abuse.

Everyday Latinx immigrants resist the institutional, systemic, and societal barriers placed before them (Arbona et al. 2010, p. 368). Gloria described using reminders of her resourcefulness in living with an undocumented immigration status to guide her in finding support, strength, well-being, and justice after experiencing sexual abuse. Like Gloria, many clients also refer to stories of their ingenuity, resourcefulness, and creativity in the face of societal barriers. When English-based characteristics, experiences, and effects of trauma are essentialized and implied as universally applicable, the realities of Spanish-speaking Latinx clients blend into a common narrative and ultimately become invisible. To interrupt these English-based trauma narratives in my work with Spanish-speaking clients, I must frequently examine the following: What implicit and explicit and essentialized English-based knowledge is accompanying the practice of translation in this organization? How does the transfer of dominant trauma narratives from the English to Spanish language influence mine and my bilingual therapist colleagues' practice of psychotherapy? How does this shape Spanish-speaking Latinx clients' experience of psychotherapy?

## Spanish Variations

The language variations of my Spanish-speaking clients are never the same. It can depend on factors such as their region, educational level, immigration status, social class, employment, or ethnicity. Spanish-speaking clients whom I consult with are immigrants of Mexican descent and other Latin American countries, like Colombia, Argentina, Guatemala, and Honduras. For some clients Spanish is their first language. For many of my indigenous clients, Spanish is a second or third language.

My own language lives in the *ni de aqui ni de alla* (from neither here nor there) of my natal Spanish and immigrant English. My Spanish originated in a small, rural, and poor agricultural town of Nayarit, Mexico, and was passed down to me by my parents. I immigrated into the English language when I entered the educational system in Escondido, CA, where decades later I also practice psychotherapy and consult with individuals and families. The city of Escondido consists of 51% Latinx individuals and 46% of homes with residents that speak a language other than English (US Census Bureau 2019). Clients and I each speak Spanish, but the sounds and expressions are different based on our singular experiences. For many clients I work with, their Spanish language has changed and evolved with life in the United States. Hence, there is less concern in the therapy room for perfection in the particularities of speaking Spanish and more consideration for how words, expressions, and phrases relate to stories of a client's life.

## A Meeting of Languages

Approaches to training and treatment at the organization position psychotherapists to identify English-based symptoms and neurobiological responses upon the first interaction with a client. Impact of Events Scale (IES)-Revised (Weiss 2007) is the required assessment to use throughout the treatment process for treatment planning and progress evaluation. It measures intrusion, avoidance, and hyperarousal symptoms that correlate with post-traumatic stress disorder. The Spanish adaptation of the IES is a direct translation of the English version.

I am vigilant for any moment when these English-based notions about the expression of trauma and understandings about psychotherapy can potentially dominate my work with Spanish-speaking Latinx clients. My stance is to maintain interest, actively and intentionally, in the clients' own language variations, experiences, understandings, and expressions and analyze throughout the therapeutic process: Am I subscribing to a translation and interpretation framework with universal assumptions about trauma in the lives of my Spanish-speaking Latinx clients? Are the client and I in a process of co-authoring with awareness about our individual Spanish variations and expressions? Am I placing judgments on my client's thoughts, emotions, and behavior or allowing clients to make judgment about trauma and its effects in their lives using their language? What is my Spanish-speaking client telling me that matters to them? Am I honoring the Spanish and language variation that the client prefers?

Spanish is invited into the session not merely as a tool that clients and I use to communicate but rather as a language and resource that can tell stories about itself and the client's experiences of trauma and psychotherapy. For instance, many Spanish-speaking Latinx clients I work with, upon initiating psychotherapy to address experiences of trauma, label the sessions as *clases*. Rather than interject with an explanation about the psychotherapy structure and act swiftly to dismiss *clases* as a cultural or linguistic misunderstanding, I inquire about how they relate psychotherapy to classes. Spanish-speaking Latinx clients I work with explain that the family court system mandated them to complete psychotherapy classes focused on learning about trauma and intimate partner violence. They express that their idea about psychotherapy or counseling *clases* is one in which they learn, as the expert psychotherapist delivers directives, advice, and direct lessons for their life. For other clients participating in psychotherapy for the first time and on a weekly basis, *clases* is the word that best reflects a similar and more familiar academic format. Some Spanish-speaking Latinx clients who have participated in prior counseling describe having experienced a teaching approach in the services they received. Those services shape their view of subsequent psychotherapy. I am interested in learning about the knowledge my Spanish-speaking clients seek for their life, which has come to motivate their desire to obtain answers about experiences of trauma.

Challenges, hopes, and aspirations after experiencing trauma are illustrated by clients I work with through Spanish language metaphors and sayings associated with their Latinx culture and language variation. When describing the effects of abuse on their behavior, sensations, thoughts, emotions, and relationships, clients may respond: it feels like the world fell upon me (*me siento como que el mundo se me vino encima*), like the world was falling from my hands (*como que el mundo se me salía de las manos*), or like the world was closing on me (*como que el mundo se me estaba cerrando*). I invite clients to expand on "experience-near" (White 2007, p. 40) descriptions using the Spanish language metaphor, or saying, that they constructed through questions such as the following: How would you describe the world that fell from your hands when you suffered abuse? What are the moments that the world seemed to be closing on you? What is the world that you speak of in that metaphor? Where inside of you do you notice the weight of the world falling upon you? How have you managed to gather the world again in your hands since experiencing trauma? Clients organize and ascribe different meanings and implications to the Spanish language variation of their metaphor. They may use it to share their present experience with powerlessness, isolation, fatigue, or preoccupation. Other clients I work with may elicit the metaphor to represent their journey and particular effects of intimate partner violence or sexual abuse that now live in the past.

## Final Reflections

Resisting the pull of dominant trauma narratives, as well as translation and interpreting notions in my psychotherapy work, is a recent undertaking. There was a point when using my bilingualism for translation and interpreting felt as advocacy for my Latinx Spanish-speaking community. Working in the field of domestic violence and sexual assault has led me to confront that translating and interpreting can function as a validation of English-based knowledge systems. The process to arrive at these observations has dismantled the ideas I once had about translation and interpretation and laid the groundwork for my own therapeutic strategies for therapeutic work that acknowledges a client's Spanish language variations, cultures, and sociopolitical issues.

## References

Arbona, C., Olvera, N., Rodriguez, N., Hagan, J., Linares, A., & Wiesner, M. (2010). Acculturative stress among documented and undocumented Latino immigrants in the United States. *Hispanic Journal of Behavioral Sciences, 32*(3), 362–384.

Bohan, J. (1993). Essentialism, constructionism, and feminist psychology. *Psychology of Women Quarterly, 17*(1), 5–21.

U.S. Census Bureau. (2019). Quick facts, Escondido. Retrieved from https://www.census.gov/quickfacts/escondidocitycalifornia.

Van der Kolk, B. A. (2014). *The body keeps the score: Brain, mind, and body in the healing of trauma*. New York: Viking.

Weiss, D. S. (2007). The impact of event scale: Revised. In J. P. Wilson & C. S. Tang (Eds.), *Cross-cultural assessment of psychological trauma and PTSD* (International and Cultural Psychology Series). Boston: Springer. https://doi.org/10.1007/978-0-387-70990-1_10.
White, M. (2007). *Maps of narrative practice*. New York: W W Norton & Co.
White, M., & Epston, D. (1990). *Narrative means to therapeutic ends*. New York, NY: W.W. Norton & Company, Inc.

# Chapter 9
# Spanish-English Bilingual Supervision

**Blanca Lizbeth Lugo**

**Abstract** Practicing Spanish-English bilingual supervision takes place in a multicultural space in which relational meanings heighten complexities of sexuality, spirituality, class, gender, and race, in the back and forth, in creation and recreation of language. Language in therapy is not detached from identity, meaning development, and worldview. Being bilingual is not just a language issue: it is a worldview, a practice, and a way of being. This chapter will discuss the motivation to become a Spanish-English bilingual supervisor, define Spanish-English bilingual supervision and my supervisor role, address the supervision language and clinical alterations, and discuss the role of social justice in bilingual supervision.

Spanish-English bilingual supervision takes place in a multicultural space in which relational meanings bring up heightened complexities of sexuality, spirituality, class, gender, and race, in the back and forth, in creation and recreation of language. Being bilingual is not just a language issue: it is a worldview, a practice, and a way of being. I am a Mexican, light-skinned, heterosexual, middle-class Spanish-English bilingual marriage and family therapist, a woman of color who literally moves between geographically constructed borders (Tijuana-San Diego) and other borders. I practice in San Diego, CA, where a great number of mental health consumers from Latin America and its diverse cultures speak Spanish.

I tailor my supervision and make alterations to better suit the needs of Spanish-speaking bilingual students. It seems likely that bilingual supervisors and therapists who speak languages other than Spanish-English may have similar experiences as the ones described in this chapter. Since my professional and language abilities are limited to Spanish-English bilingualism, I will focus only on my experiences as a Spanish-English bilingual therapist and supervisor. In this chapter, I will discuss my experience of becoming a Spanish-English bilingual supervisor, define my supervisory role, and address linguistic, clinical, and cultural alterations to supervision. Due to the dearth of studies examining the various dimensions of Spanish-English

B. L. Lugo (✉)
Private Practice, San Diego State University, San Diego, CA, USA



m. polanco et al. (eds.), *Bilingualism, Culture, and Social Justice in Family Therapy*, AFTA SpringerBriefs in Family Therapy,
https://doi.org/10.1007/978-3-030-66036-9_9

bilingual supervision, this chapter offers an accounting of the literature and my own experiences in training, ongoing consultation, and experimenting with trainees from a stance of responsible curiosity.

## Becoming a Spanish-English Bilingual Supervisor

In my practicum and traineeship experiences, I attended programs that offered live supervision. I had one bilingual English/Spanish supervisor who understood the content of my conversations with clients, but I was unable to learn from my monolingual English-speaking peers' feedback. I was ill-prepared to apply the knowledge I had received in English from my training program to provide supervision to Spanish-English bilingual students, just as I was ill-prepared to apply learned theory and interventions in Spanish and with the Latinx community.

After becoming licensed, I assisted a practicum class as a translator for a monolingual English-speaking supervisor. I witnessed the limited supervision that the only Spanish-English bilingual student received when having me as a behind the mirror translator for her live supervision sessions. I realized then that other therapists in training were experiencing a similar predicament to the one I experienced in my training and recognized that Spanish-speaking clients often get low-quality services under such therapists in training; so I decided to become a supervisor in hopes I could work toward bridging the gap of quality services for the Latinx community.

I began teaching a practicum class at a couple of San Diego, CA, local marriage and family therapy (MFT) master's level programs. Some of the students in the first cohorts expressed feeling comfortable with their Spanish and English language skills and thus were requested by their training programs to serve Latinx clients who were monolingual Spanish speakers. In those beginning stages of my supervisory development, I understood that students' struggles were much like the ones I had experienced years before: they had inadequate access to appropriate training, and there was limited literature on working with monolingual Spanish Latinx clients.

A great majority of Spanish-English bilingual mental health professionals have identified not receiving linguistically appropriate training to serve the Latinx population (Trepal et al. 2014; Valencia-García and Montoya 2018). The limited research on this issue identifies bilingual supervision as key in learning how to serve the Latinx population and in increasing the students' confidence in their own psychotherapeutic skills (Valencia-García and Montoya 2018). Usually, bilingual students seek literature, consultation, and supervision on their own (Trepal et al. 2014). To access Spanish-English supervision has been as challenging to students as accessing mental health services has been for Latinx consumers (Trepal et al. 2014; Valencia-García and Montoya 2018).

The challenges for many of my Spanish-English bilingual students involve limited resources and affirming supervision relationships, as well as ethnocentricity and racism that permeate education institutions in which we are only visible if we adapt to a White middle-class Eurocentric paradigm. MFT Spanish-English bilingual students experience questioning from faculty and peers, opposition, and dismissal when voicing a need for linguistically and culturally appropriate training to serve the Latinx community in San Diego.

For example, some faculty members once responded to my students' feedback by including one invited guest to address in a few hours theoretical cultural and linguistic applications for Spanish-English bilingual students. However, when students continued requesting additional training, they were labeled as demanding and entitled.

Few years ago, access to additional training and Spanish-English bilingual supervision was advocated by some of the bilingual students and was finally granted by the educational institution. Some non-bilingual (monolingual English-speaking) students expressed disapproval and opposition to Spanish-English bilingual students receiving access to bilingual supervision, and they accused their program directors of providing special treatment for Spanish-English supervision. They openly referred to the Spanish-English bilingual student practicum group as the "Mexican Lab." Validating and channeling students' experiences of racism and discrimination has been an integral part of my role as a Spanish-English bilingual supervisor, a role that will be further addressed in this chapter.

## Spanish-English Supervision

González et al. (2015) defined bilingual supervision as occurring when "one member of the client-counselor-supervisor triad is communicating primarily in a language other than English" (p.185). However, I contend that bilingual supervision is also multicultural supervision; it involves deconstruction and reconstruction of realities and relationships. Language in therapy is in the body: we feel it; it narrates the stories of our lives. It is not detached from what matters to us.

### *Spanish-English Supervisor Role*

As an MFT Spanish-English bilingual supervisor, I have often been a language broker between my students and the mental health professional community. I act as a bridge between two contexts: the therapeutic relationship with their Latinx clients and the Eurocentric context of the mental health profession.

I use the concept and experiences of bilingualism as an analogy to teach students about the relationship between the culturally and linguistically appropriate services they aim to render to their Latinx clients and the clinical and professional expectations of Eurocentric places of work. From case conceptualization formats to clinical documentation guidelines, my role is to speak and translate such languages in the hopes that they will soon feel comfortable working toward proficiency in both languages.

My supervisory role also includes engaging in conversations regarding contextual variables with the purpose of exploring the students' racial and language identities and the dominant discourses that have informed them (Hernández 2003; Taylor et al. 2006). I am responsible, when conversing about racial and language identities, to support and mentor the healing process from the macroaggressions they have experienced. Students learn to reframe their oppressive experiences as windows into the oppression that clients often experience when attempting to access mental health services. This also allows students to explore their role as agents of social change within the mental health professional field (González et al. 2015).

## *Supervision Alterations*

To address the training needs of Spanish-English bilingual students, I modified the process of clinical supervision to include attention to language and clinical alterations.

### Language Alterations

Delgado-Romero et al. (2018) explain that part of the role of a Spanish-English bilingual mental health provider is to be a language broker. As a Spanish-English supervisor, I am a language broker. I attempt to bridge my Spanish-speaking students with the mainstream culture of mental health academia and professions. My language brokering process includes exploring the student's comfort of their perceived Spanish proficiency, identifying mental health Spanish vocabulary, and translating theory and interventions.

#### Student's Language Proficiency Comfort

Many students who express interest in serving the Latinx community also express concerns about their linguistic ability to serve monolingual Spanish clients (Estrada et al. 2018; Trepal et al. 2014). Thus, the first step in the Spanish-English supervision process has been to engage in a conversation around language proficiency comfort. Students often have a diverse range of acculturation experiences that influence their perception of their language proficiency skills.

As a Spanish-English bilingual supervisor, I utilize this conversation as a port of entry to begin building a non-judgmental clinical supervisory relationship. I honor the students' comfort level and their decisions to either begin rendering mental health services in Spanish, to engage in further learning of Spanish language, or to shadow other students with different levels of language proficiency and comfort. The comfort of Spanish-English bilingual students, as probably many other bilingual students, around usage of a second language might differ based mainly on their perception of language proficiency skills. I provide psychoeducation on the disparity of quality services the Latinx community experiences (Delgado-Romero et al. 2018) to encourage students in becoming agents of social change by closing that gap, and I share experiences in navigating linguistic challenges.

### Spanish Mental Health Vocabulary

Since the great majority of students receive mental health training in English, Spanish mental health vocabulary proficiency is a challenge for all regardless of overall Spanish language proficiency comfort level. There are some published resources that can help students begin to become familiar with Spanish mental health terminology (Bender et al. 2006; Gutierrez et al. 2010), but often students have collaborated in developing their own tools (such as a glossary) that fit their personal comfort levels and their client's Spanish language proficiencies.

I have been a witness to how the Latinx collectivistic culture manifests in MFT practicum cohorts where students collaborate and share identified and developed resources. My role is to identify and reflect those cultural dynamics that can be applied to their therapeutic relationships with Latinx clients. I share with them that their collaboration in developing Spanish-English students' group tools can be utilized as a clinical intervention by collaborating with their clients in identifying useful resources and tools to assist clients and their communities.

## Clinical Alterations

MFT Spanish-English bilingual students are expected to perform many additional processes compared to their monolingual peers. Bilingual students must learn theoretical knowledge in English and then translate, adjust, and apply the knowledge into Spanish. They must learn to adapt, adjust, and apply mainstream knowledge about mental health into the Latinx culture. They must translate the session process and content back into English, as well as adapt, adjust, and apply the session process and content onto mainstream theoretical concepts and academic assessment of their skills (González et al. 2015). In order to assist the laborious process described above, I focus on two main areas: translating theory and interventions and enhancing the clinical interventions learned primarily for their use with English-speaking clients.

## Translating Theory and Interventions

Assisting students in the translation of theoretical concepts into Spanish and the Latinx culture has been the most challenging and delicate dance of the Spanish-English supervision process. I believe that if we are to be efficient in rendering services to Spanish monolingual clients, it is key that we converse about a clinical case in the client's spoken language. If the client is monolingual Spanish, it is recommended to only utilize Spanish during our clinical discussion (González et al. 2015).

Once the client's language is identified for purposes of case presentation, the MFT student can identify the theory of therapy to which she/he/they feel(s) most inclined. We can then engage in a conversation about the theory's epistemology, as well as the client's cultural epistemology. Thereafter, we can discuss what would be an appropriate theoretical translation of theory into the client's Spanish. A similar process is followed for interventions; we engage in a conversation about the goals of interventions, how will they be adapted into Spanish, and the risks of literal translations.

### Clinical Intervention Alterations

Fortunately, there are great Latinx authors who have addressed the need to integrate a cultural lens into interventions and treatment approaches. These authors have emphasized the need to consider the interplay of communication styles, gender dynamics, spirituality, immigration, etc., and how these variables differ from mainstream White American culture (Comas-Díaz and Greene 1994; Espín 1997; Falicov 1998). Role-play is utilized to practice the cultural and linguistic adaptation of interventions. Collaborative feedback also models culturally and linguistically appropriate conversations that can be transferred from the supervision room into the therapy room. Conversations during supervision are focused on addressing and acknowledging the various cultural dynamics played in the relationships between peers, between student group and supervisor, and between individuals in the collective of practicum group and supervisor.

## Cultural Alterations

I weave cultural alterations in supervisory interaction. The cultural lens is embedded in every aspect, including identification of our cultural locations, collaboratively determining class structure, sharing of the food and beverages during supervision sessions, and the celebration of supervision relationship termination (Falicov 1998; Hernández 2003; Taylor et al. 2006). I utilize communication styles common in Latinx culture such as using *dichos*, discussions on appropriateness of language terms such as *usted* vs. *tu*, and reflection on the cultural language of externalization of locus of control, etc. (Falicov 1998). Ignoring cultural nuances when addressing the mental health of individuals from marginalized populations can further perpetuate oppression. Thus, to not assess, mold, and polish these cultural alterations would be a tremendous ethical violation (Hernández 2003; Taylor et al. 2006; Trepal et al. 2014; Valencia-García and Montoya 2018).

## Socially Just Supervision

Cultural humility shines a light onto the many theoretical limitations in clinical practice that arise when working with clients who have lived in marginalized communities (Fuertes 2004). Thus, as it has been the case in my work, cultural humility could provide mental health professionals, including MFT Spanglish-English bilingual students with a framework to recognize the training, theoretical, and research limitations that inform their work and to form collaborations with clients to identify and polish successful interventions. As a supervisor, I must practice what I preach. This means I must continually consult, re-define, polish, adapt, and adjust collaboratively with those that I supervise. I recognize I have limited access to training and research on how to optimally provide Spanish-English bilingual supervision. Thus, it is my responsibility to ensure that through collaboration, I can work to balance the power I hold as a representative of the Eurocentric mental health profession and Eurocentric mental health training institution or agency (Delgado-Romero et al. 2018).

## Conclusion

In this chapter, I discussed experiences around the process of becoming a Spanish-English bilingual supervisor, how clinical supervision of Spanish-English bilingual MFT students has included language, clinical, and cultural alterations. I have also outlined how I define my role as an ethically responsible Spanish-English bilingual supervisor to include adapting, supporting, advocating, and encouraging power-balanced relationships for Spanish-English bilingual students and their Latinx clients.

Linguistically and ethnically diverse students are deserving of culturally and linguistically humble supervisors, just as clients are deserving of linguistically humble psychotherapists. As MFT educators and supervisors, we cannot continue to ignore the role bilingualism plays in the collaborative process of developing meaning, trust, confidence, and skills for the psychotherapeutic process. We must acknowledge that languages other than English are to be honored as a key contextual variable if our goal is truly successful psychotherapist development.

## References

Bender, D. E., Harlan, C., Ko, L., & Stern, I. (2006). *Spanish for mental health professionals: A step by step handbook*. Albuquerque: University of New Mexico Press.

Comas-Díaz, L., & Greene, B. A. (1994). *Women of color: Integrating ethnic and gender identities in psychotherapy*. New York: Guilford Publications.

Delgado-Romero, E. A., De los Santos, J., Raman, V., Merrifield, J., Vázquez, M., Cárdenas Bautista, E., & Duran, M. Y. (2018). Caught in the middle: Spanish-speaking bilingual mental health counselors as language brokers. *Journal of Mental Health Counseling, 40*(4), 341–352. https://doi.org/10.17744/melgc.40.4.06.

Espín, O. (1997). *Latina realities: Essays on healing, migration, and sexuality*. New York: Routledge.

Estrada, O., Brown, J. L. C., & Molloy, L. (2018). Bilingual therapists' confidence using clinical Spanish language terminology. *Journal of Teaching in Social Work, 38*(3), 324–341. https://doi.org/10.1080/08841233.2018.1468384.

Falicov, C. J. (1998). *Latino families in therapy: A guide to multicultural practice*. New York: The Guilford Press.

Fuertes, J. (2004). Supervision in bilingual counseling: Services delivery, training, and research considerations. *Journal of Multicultural Counseling and Development, 32*, 84–94.

González, L. M., Ivers, N. N., Noyola, M. C., Murillo-Herrera, A. C., & Davis, K. M. (2015). Supervision in Spanish: Reflections from supervisor-trainee dyads. *The Clinical Supervisor, 34*, 184–203. https://doi.org/10.1080/07325223.2015.1058208.

Gutierrez, V., Rafiee, C., Bartelma, E. K., & Guerra, V. (2010). *An English-Spanish manual for mental health professionals*. San Diego: CreateSpace Independent Publishing Platform.

Hernández, P. (2003). The cultural context model in supervision: An illustration. *Journal of Feminist Family Therapy, 15*(4), 1–18. https://doi.org/10.1300/J086v15n04_01.

Taylor, B. A., Hernández, P., Deri, A., Ranking, I. P. R., & Siegel, A. (2006). Integrating diversity dimensions in supervision: Perspectives of ethnicity minority AAMFT approved supervisors. *Clinical Supervisor, 25*(1/2), 3–21. https://doi.org/10.1300/J001v25n01-02.

Trepal, H., Ivers, N., & Lopez, A. (2014). Students' experiences with bilingual counseling. *The Journal of Counselor Preparation and Supervision, 6*(2). https://doi.org/10.7729/62.1096.

Valencia-García, D., & Montoya, H. (2018). Lost in translation: Training issues for bilingual students in health service psychology. *Training and Education in Professional Psychology, 12*(3), 142–148. https://doi.org/10.1037/tep0000199.

# Chapter 10
# Legitimizing Language Traffick(ing) Through a Community of Support

**Mu-Lan Chau, Letti Estrella, Ingrid Guerrieri, and Daniel O'Sullivan**

**Abstract** In this chapter, we tell our stories as four bilingual Latin American marriage and family therapists (MFTs) who have been coming together to form a community of support. Our stories highlight the complexities of providing therapeutic services in a language different from that of our training and the mainstream understandings of bilingual clinical work. The chapter illustrates how the work developed in our collaborative community has helped legitimize the unconventional ways in which we practice. Individual narratives provide examples of clinical language and therapeutic practices, which include language traffick(ing), *palabras de a centavo* and *terapia de la calle*. Our hope in contributing this chapter is to expand the field's interest in the topic of therapy in languages other than English.

This is a telling about the experience of four Latin American bilingual – Spanish and English – marriage and family therapists (MFTs) who have been coming together to form a community of support. *Las comadres*, as we affectionately have come to call ourselves, meet biweekly to discuss the complexities of working in a language that is outside of the cultural mainstream and that is different from the one in which we learned our trade and our clinical training. We work in San Diego, California, a city that shares the international border with Tijuana, Baja California, and rests upon the traditional and unceded land of the Kumeyaay Nation. This territory bears the legacy of scars and wounds inflicted through centuries of territorial, linguistic, and cultural pillage and is defined today by the constant transborder

M. Chau (✉)
Associate Marriage and Family Therapist, Riverside, CA, USA

L. Estrella
SDSU Center for Community Counseling and Engagement CCCE, SDSU Centro de Consejería para la Comunidad CCCE, San Diego, CA, USA

I. Guerrieri
Christie's Place, San Diego, CA, USA

D. O'Sullivan
Narrative Initiatives of San Diego, San Diego, CA, USA



m. polanco et al. (eds.), *Bilingualism, Culture, and Social Justice in Family Therapy*, AFTA SpringerBriefs in Family Therapy,
https://doi.org/10.1007/978-3-030-66036-9_10

traffic of people, goods, and narratives where linguistic and cultural identities are in constant flux and negotiation.

Like our clients, *no somos ni de aquí ni de allá* – we are neither local nor fully outsiders. Wittgenstein (1922) wrote that "the limits of my language means the limits of my world" (p.74). This holds true for us. Language both restricts and expands the edges of our experience of the world. Our worlds were "languaged" at first, in Chilean, Colombian, and Mexican Spanish; now they must be continually constructed in a Spanish that has been influenced by English and all sorts of Spanish. Our work therefore was born by choice and necessity, between the territories covered by and constructed in two languages, traffick(ing) across words, identities, and meaning making. It explores and calls attention to the cartographical multilayering of our sociopolitical, geographical, linguistic, and affective landscape.

While the focus of this chapter is on language, it also aims to document a specific kind of positioning and relational engagement that invites the knowledge of our *ancestros*, the idiosyncrasies of our *tierra(s)*, and the complex realities of our current sociopolitical contexts, practices that seem non-conventional and that became possible only through the legitimizing effects of engaging in a community of support.

We defy the widely held notion that working with transcultural populations is simply a matter of translation and that translation equates to language substitution. In our practice, we do a different kind of "translating" where languages are combined, Spanglish, and/or alternated, code switching, as means to honor and expand the knowledge and skills of our clients. To us, language substitution is a perilous oversimplification that marginalizes such knowledge and skills. It is akin to working under a sort of free trade agreement (FTA), a system that, by streamlining tariffs and duties, is, in theory, supposed to reduce barriers and benefit all parties equally but that in reality creates new forms of disparity and exploitation.

In our experience, monocultural therapists – informed by mainstream assumptions about mental health, the traditional role of the therapists and patients, and psychotherapy as a practice – tend to misread our work as chaotic and illegitimate, rather than clinical. We chose to embrace these misreadings when we named our practices "language traffick(ing)." Our individual voices coalesce below, around the notion of language traffick(ing), as well as its micro applications, such as *palabras de a centavo* and *terapia de la calle.*

## Mu-Lan

*Esta chilena* joined las *comadres* in 2018, at the start of my MFT training. As any other budding therapist who is just getting to do some work with clients, I was nervous and full of questions yet excited about having the chance to serve the Spanish speaking community. I was under the impression that I would be able to simply apply the knowledge from my classes with all my clients, as if I had signed a sort of FTA agreement, but soon realized that passage in the territories of language is not as free and smooth as I imagined. New-therapist fears gave way to other insecurity-inducing feelings as I realized I would also have to figure out how to apply my training in English to my practice in Spanish. I felt overwhelmed but found with *las comadres* a space for curiosity, vulnerability, open discussion, and a genuine willingness for support.

I consider *comadre* conversations to constitute a significant part of my training as a therapist. In the group, I have the chance to question and try out my understanding of theoretical, cultural, and linguistic aspects of my work without judgment. All the other *comadres* are further along in their professional development; nonetheless my questions are accepted and the group engages with them in ways that make me feel like a contributor; this has encouraged me to be present with all parts of me: my Chilean *palabras de a centavo* – Chilean Spanish colloquialisms, playfulness, and my interest in bringing in and integrating my artist identity to my clinical work.

Though I continue to introduce some invitations and ideas in therapy as *raras* (weird) or crazy, I know I am confident in the knowledge that, when listening and sharing perspectives in therapy, I am actively and intentionally engaging in traffick(ing), rather than smuggling. *Comadre* conversations make it possible for me to experience my work with a sense of wonder, as feeling connected and supported allows creativity and intuition to join me in the room. In the group I have come to understand that I struggled to ask what in translation would result in weird-sounding questions, because providing care in Spanish requires bringing in additional and unusual resources.

The collaborative and non-hierarchical dynamics in the group have been invaluable in my ability to move away from insecurity and fear. Working in this way invites centering of the personal and collective aspects of ancestral wisdom and cultural heritage(s) present in the bilingual and bicultural aspects of our experience. Being a *comadre* has provided a context of legitimization and inclusion and an invitation into creative explorations of my linguistic and relational approach to therapy.

## Letti

A brown woman, a Mexican *migrante* from Veracruz – a *Jarocha*. For me, speaking in simple terms is a personal and intentional choice made as I found literal translation constituted an insufficient rendering for someone else's message. Upon arrival to the USA, I was entrusted by family and neighbors with the task of interpreting the language and customs of our new country – this is my first experience in language and cultural brokerage.

Traffick(ing) with words, for me, invites the use of colloquial language, *palabras de a centavo*, a language that is deeply rooted in the mannerisms of *mi pueblo's* dialect and my *Jarocha* identity – informal, *dicharachero* language that communicates ancestral wisdom in welcoming and funny ways. It sounds unpretentious, authentic, and playful; it inspires trust and leaves aside suspicion.

In colloquial *Jarocha* language, the phrase *no vale un centavo* denotes insignificant value, and so these *palabras* seen through the gaze of the colonizing "proper" Castilian Spanish have little value and are therefore unwelcomed in professional and academic settings, yet they are naturally welcomed in therapeutic conversations. Because of my history as a linguistic and cultural broker, I entered the helping professions planning to continue traffick(ing) with colloquial vocabularies in therapy, yet I always felt I *was* doing something *illegal*; I felt isolated and afraid someone would find out I was engaging in such "illicit" activity – using language that was poor and informal.

Joining a group of colleagues who question the mainstreamed idea of therapy with whom I share the hope of delivering unconventional therapeutic practice opened opportunities for co-creating a space of support and holding one another in our clinical work. These conversations have "legalized" the way in which I position myself and traffic language in the therapeutic room. During group discussions about the influences of English in our training and the complexities and different implications of the work that we do in *Español*, I felt safe. I confessed my crime to the group: traffick(ing) and smuggling *palabras de a centavo* in therapy. I introduced it as a therapeutic practice influenced by my childhood's "unconventional translating" experience and by my own quotidian, accessible Spanish. Borrowing from my client's colloquialisms and my own linguistic background helps me level the hierarchical authority within the therapeutic relationship, leaves out formality, and evokes a sense of trust among therapist and client. It helps one to feel relaxed and particularly avoids making one feeling judged linguistically. This language traffick(ing) was welcomed in our conversations, and it contributed to discussions of additional unconventional ways of translating that facilitate and in a way legalize the language that we as bilingual therapists use.

Today, as an MFT, a professional linguistic authority still forces me to continue traffick(ing) language while working with those who often speak colloquial Spanish. I invite *palabras de a centavo* knowing that, for my clients, this "cheap" language connects and has worth. Adopting my ancestors' wisdom in the form of sayings such as *Crea fama y echate a dormir* into a therapy session to express a loss of trust, for example, can provide a deeper sense of understanding and solidarity. Similarly, I also use phrases such as "it sounds as if you were eating a taco *sin aguacate*" to highlight in a non-critical voice that a member of a family is not fully satisfied with an explanation they are hearing. I use *palabras de a centavo* because it sounds modest, genuine, and playful. It inspires confidence and leaves aside suspicion, all producing effects that allow for a special and relational way of engaging.

## Ingrid

*Terapia de la calle* is what I have come to call my ways of relating in my therapist role. The name came about during *comadre* conversations, as our confessing to not abiding by the normative standards of the clinical counseling field prompted discussions about how code switching one's way through clinical interventions does not constitute an appropriate approach to bilingual work. Let me illustrate with some *terapia de la calle* examples.

Interactions in my therapeutic work take place in Mexican, Colombian, and borderland Spanish, which invites considerations of the effects of languaging and meaning making in the relational dynamic. *Terapia de la calle* invites paying attention to the worlds all of these *Españoles* make possible: from delineating social positioning to literal and figurative meanings of words and expressions. My clients and I are actively involved in clarification and questioning of assumptions, like the time when a Chicano client and I realized we were formulating goals for therapy under contradictory appreciations of his story. The problem resided in that, while I was encouraging him to ally with *coraje* (bravery) in his dealing with depression, he found *coraje* (anger) to be a fervent proponent of resentment and stagnation. Sometimes the Colombian meaning does not match the Mexican or Chicano definition of a term, in addition to the frequent calques from English that emerge in the borderland; here the carpet is a *carpeta*, which in Colombia is a folder, and a truck is a *troca*, which to a Colombian is bartering.

Another significant aspect of my practice as *terapia de la calle* is the political implications of language; using clinical or academic language invites hierarchical positioning between therapist and client, which determines who we are and what is possible for each of us in the relationship. I actively consult, and mostly abide, by clients' preference on how they want to be addressed yet subvert the assumed power differential in the relationship by intentionally smuggling words and expressions from my Colombian Spanish. While at the beginning of therapy I use formal epithets such as *sumercé*, *usted*, and *mi señora*, I soon move toward *mijo* and *mamasita* to increase a sense of intimacy; I also use *doctora* to emphasize their role as contributors and partners. I find that it is easier for people to allow me to use *mamasita* or *doctora* before consenting to using the informal form of you (*tú*), as the former expressions are taken to be a Colombian thing rather than an overt challenge to the assumed hierarchical order.

*Terapia de la calle* links language usage to the spatial, somatic, and relational aspects of the therapy session with intentionality. Negotiating and tending to the relationship can include organizing furniture as a living room and inviting clients to try out different chairs or sit on the floor, discussing consent around hugs and greeting/departure rituals, and sharing food or a hot beverage. It is through ethically and clinically informed uses of my Colombianness that language supports me in creating intimacy and trust, making it possible to experience the work as an afternoon *cafecito* in any space, even when telling painful stories. *Terapia de la calle* describes a relational practice, an intentional way of being and doing, enacted through language.

Before engaging in curiosity-driven inquiry with my *comadres*, my sharing of *terapia de la calle* was met with criticism. It became legitimized as reflections in the group highlighted the false assumptions of the bilingual FTA: that my training in English provides the cultural and linguistic resources for working competently in Spanish. I now identify as a loud-and-proud practitioner of *terapia de la calle*, knowing that, though I cannot free myself completely from the vigilant gaze of mainstream counseling, I am no longer a smuggler of illegal cargo.

## Daniel

Growing up in Colima, Mexico, I saw my father – a white American ex-pat – constantly negotiate different degrees of social membership; these were often connected to whether he was addressed by the informal pronoun *tú* or the formal *usted* or if using prefix titles, such as *Don José* or *Mister O'Sullivan*, subtle yet powerful ways to indicate levels of inclusion and of standing in a Spanish-speaking community.

As a clinician and immigrant, I have become interested in the embodied recognition, tense body and shallow breath, of being on the outside. It is a porous experience that can import indicting, prescriptive narratives such as surely, *son mis nervios* – my own anxiety – *que no?* For a social constructionist clinician, the difference between assessing otherness, as a private experience of personal deficiency (*mis nervios*) or as a publicly constructed experience of exclusion, makes all the difference in the world. Language traffick(ing) allows for the import of linguistic elements that counterweight some of the colonizing pressures and otherings that our clients face. One such linguistic practice is to pay close attention to the use of culturally significant prefixes and pronouns, elevating them both from colloquial niceties to strategic deployments of language.

In my clinical role, working for an agency contracted by our county, I received a call from a man who spoke Mexican Spanish and who had been instructed by the police department to call us. Felipe – not his real name – had reported a violent gang of faceless men trying to break into his home. Terrified by their ability to vanish when the police arrived, he was tortured by the thought of what might happen to his family should they manage to break in.

Language traffick(ing) allowed me to do three things: (1) trust that bringing in culturally relevant pronouns and prefixes, such as referring to him as *Jefe* (boss) and *Don Felipe* and asking for his permission to address him by the pronoun *tú* instead of *usted*, would have positive effects on identity construction; (2) trust that different identity states, belonging, promote different physiological states, relaxation; and (3) be on the lookout for evidence of these differences, such as pausing before answering questions, easier breathing, and a more relaxed tone of voice. Toward the end, Felipe reported that the call had not been what he expected. He described it as useful and offered a beautiful thought: perhaps he could pay attention and trust his wife's level of stress to decide whether he should be stressed at all.

## Crossing *la(s) línea(s)* with More Confidence

It is important to highlight that language traffick(ing) is an emerging practice; as you read this chapter, you are engaging with a text made possible by this unconventional way of translating. This is our English language rendering of group conversations and construction of knowledge that mostly took place in *Español(es)* and Spanglish; it relies on words and ideas that have crossed *la línea* (international border crossing) back and forth, trafficked many times.

A community of support has been imperative to help legitimize these unconventional ways of translating and engaging, and it has also made possible that we now cross the border between languages with more confidence. Our hope in contributing this chapter is to expand the field's interest in the topic of therapy in languages other than English. We are curious about the possible reflections and questions our experience may inspire in therapists who only speak English; those who work in multicultural contexts and must use translators; and those who, despite speaking other languages, do not have the chance to practice in them.

Finally, we would like to leave you with an invitation for reflection. Do you feel scrutinized or censored by prescriptive ideas about your identity and practice as a therapist? What do your language exchanges in clinical practice look like? What linguistic considerations would be helpful in engaging with the people with whom you collaborate? Is there room for language traffick(ing) in your practice? How do you imagine intentionally subversive language practices could impact the work you do in therapy? How do you imagine that engaging in your version of *terapia de la calle* and *palabras de a centavo* would impact your clients' and your experience in therapy? Who are the people in your world that share some of your worldview and could become your collaborators or fellow language traffickers? We are convinced we are not alone in our thirst for collaboration and support and hope you find yourself in a community of *comadres* soon.

## Reference

Wittgenstein, L. (1922). *Tractatus Logico-Philosophicus*. New York: Harcourt, Brace & Company.

# Chapter 11
# Corazones Bilingües: A Journey in MFT Training and Practice

**Rocio Ocampo-Giancola, Gricelda Alvarez, and Elvia Murga**

**Abstract** During our marriage and family training, we have often navigated between Pocho *Spanish*, *Spanglish*, *Spanish* only, and other forms of language negotiation. We have utilized a diverse set of linguistic skills in almost every session with the clients whose *historias* we witnessed and participated in. In this chapter, we reflect on the effects of internalized shame, language barriers, advocacy, language discrimination, and racism in our personal and professional lives as marriage and family therapists working with *Spanish*-speaking families from a social justice ethics in Southern California. We explore how our *corazones bilingües* are guided by language and identify the need for language proficiency training in our field and in MFT graduate programs.

> Until I am free to write bilingually and to switch codes without having to always translate, while I still have to speak English or Spanish when I would rather speak Spanglish, as long as I have to accommodate the English speakers rather than having them accommodate me, my tongue will be illegitimate. I will no longer be made to feel ashamed for existing. I will have my voice: Indian, Spanish, White. I will have my serpents tongue….I will overcome the tradition of silence. (Anzaldúa 1999, p. 81)

Our goal in writing this chapter is to bring to light the lack of training for marriage and family bilingual clinicians and the anti-immigration views that surround us and to discuss language and its impact in our own lives. Throughout our MFT training and practice, we have often used Pocho Spanish, Spanglish, Spanish only, and English. Pocho Spanish refers to an Americanized Spanish influenced by the English language, while Spanglish is a hybrid language made up of both English and Spanish words intertwined. In our experiences, the Pocho Spanish and even Spanglish are often seen as less than and critiqued as "less educated." For us, it is crucial to acknowledge that these kinds of beliefs are at the root of the language discrimination and division that exists in our communities. Becoming aware of how we, three first-generation Mexican bilingual clinicians, understand language as fluid

R. Ocampo-Giancola (✉)
Private Practice, San Diego, CA, USA

G. Alvarez · E. Murga
San Diego, CA, USA



m. polanco et al. (eds.), *Bilingualism, Culture, and Social Justice in Family Therapy*, AFTA SpringerBriefs in Family Therapy,
https://doi.org/10.1007/978-3-030-66036-9_11

rather than static and a cultural construct, a process, has and continues to impact us as individuals and clinicians.

In 2016, we had the privilege of collaborating together while working with the Latinx community, primarily Mexican community, in San Diego, California, during a time when there was increased anti-immigrant sentiment and draconian immigrant policies throughout the United States. Gricelda questioned therapy theories that she did not feel translated to the work she was doing with her clients marginalized by language, poverty, and language issues. Elvia worked at a school setting predominantly with bilingual children crossing the border or recently immigrated to the United States. She was navigating a school administrator imposing "English-only counseling sessions." A student that was referred to her was relieved that she could speak in Spanish while in session with her. We listened to our *corazones*, holding higher our ethics for people's right to use their language than the English-only rules. Rocio worked in an immigration detention center that held undocumented immigrant women and children from San Martin Peras, Oaxaca, Central and South America. Narrative therapy ideas such as the role of "non-expert" and that "people are not passive in the face of trauma" informed her practice in therapy and supervision (White 2006). In the next couple of pages, we urge you to listen to your *corazón* as you join us in our journey and bear witness to our realizations.

## *¿A ti quién te soporta*?/Who Tolerates You? *Eso no suena bien*

My name is Gricelda Alvarez. At the beginning of my first marriage and family therapist (MFT) practicum, in San Diego, California, I witnessed how using Spanglish, the mixing of English and Spanish words to communicate with Latinx clients, frequently interrupted the initial rapport between a non-native Spanish mental health provider and the Latinx client(s). The following is how I experienced, translated, and weaved my Mexican culture throughout my MFT practicum experience, a field primarily immersed as much today as yesterday in the dominant discourse where compliance is still a must for one to move on.

While I was trained by a leading non-native Spanish marriage and family therapist in a clinical site where we mostly assisted monolingual Spanish Latinx client(s), I recognized that the way the clinicians asked the Latinx clients *¿a ti quién te soporta*?/who tolerates you? *No sonaba bien*/did not sound right. It often triggered a visible upset reaction among some monolingual Spanish-speaking clients leaving them feeling offended, confused, and disrespected. Even though it was a required question to complete the client's initial intake, the sound of the question *¿a ti quién te soporta*? was not always welcome.

Rightfully so, because they were hearing the literal translation and not what the clinician thought they were hearing, who is your support group?/*¿quién es tu grupo de apoyo*? Unfortunately, for the Latinx families, that was not it. Sadly, the rapport of the moment got lost in the lit*eral Spanglish tra*nslation. Thus, the client ended up hearing *¿a ti quién te soporta?*/who tolerates you? The sound of the words support/

soporta somehow sounded similar to the non-native Spanish mental health provider. After all, this is something understandable, since the sounds of words like beard, beer, saw, and I saw, for the most part, sounded the same to this Mexican in her first English class. Nonetheless, each holds a different meaning.

Although I realized the question the monolingual clinician asked the client *no sonaba bien*/did not sound right to a monolingual Spanish-speaking client, I stayed quiet. At that moment, I did not feel there was a choice for me. After all, I was the MFT trainee. I did not want to undermine my peer and I also wanted to respect the clients' right to advocate for themselves. Some of the clients asked the clinician to explain why they were asked that question. It did not make sense to them. As a bilingual, native speaker in Spanish did not make sense to me either. It was from this practicum experience that I began to fully understand the assertion made by Santiago-Rivera and Altarriba (2002) on how "language in therapy is central to effective treatment regardless of theoretical orientation" (p.30).

After much reflection, Santiago-Rivera and Altarriba (2002) inspired me to think about my professional responsibility to the Spanish monolingual Latinx community. I became mindful of Spanglish words' power to avoid offending clients and prevent losing them in their first therapy session; more so, knowing that the therapeutic process and alliance begins from the first point of contact with the client. Furthermore, I noticed that, for the brave Latinx families who mustered the courage to tolerate/*soportar* the stigma and shame of seeking mental health services, they regularly found themselves lost in literal translations. More efforts are necessary for language competency to minimize Spanglish incongruities, for once the monolingual Latinx's client heard the dissonance of the statement, the client(s) were left feeling unsupported, misunderstood, and or disrespected.

Aguilar-Gaxiola et al.' (2012) research concluded that several factors (i.e., language, legal, financial) continue to influence the mental health services offered to the Latinx community and that "ineffective communication between provider and patient" (p. 2) is one of the main reasons for low rates of mental health access and retention. It is up to me and the MFT field to make the best efforts to practice language with humility and recognize that the Latinx community goes against all the odds and stigma of *estas loco* to show up for their therapy sessions. Clients' courage to show up benefits me because it allows me to master my clinical skills and eventually allows many clinicians to obtain their licenses. For me clients deserve respect and, at a minimum, language proficiency from the providers. In order to fulfill this need for language proficiency, graduate MFT's programs need to include language proficiency throughout the program.

## *¿Qué hago?* Unlearning Shame

In 2003 when I was 8 years old, I, Elvia Murga, immigrated to the United States from Mexicali, B.C., and quickly realized that my Spanish was not welcomed here. Teachers at school scolded me when I would speak Spanish, *tienes que hablar inglés* they would say, and my peers always seemed to laugh when I spoke in class. These negative experiences left me spending my first few years in the United States trying to eradicate *mi acento*, an accent so telling that it always reminds others *qué yo no soy de aquí*. It is now 2020 and after 17 years of living in the United States, *mi corazón* still feels in Spanish.

I began my journey as an MFT graduate student in May 2016 at San Diego State University, where I would spend 2 years participating in discussions about diversity, social justice, and cultural competence. As I began working with bilingual and monolingual *Spanish*-speaking individuals and families, it quickly became apparent that something *no estaba bien*. The skills, theories, and ideas I had spent hours learning and practicing in English were somehow not translating into the work with *mi gente*. *No se sentia bien*. I began to bring my concerns to my Anglo-speaking professors who did not adequately address my questions from their English vantage point. I was left confused; I began to feel isolated and I asked myself *¿Soy yo?*

In my quest for answers, I discovered a book titled *The Borderlands/La frontera* by Gloria Anzaldúa (1999). *Mi corazón bilingüe* connected to her stories of the in-betweenness and feeling forced to pick one language when navigating a world of many (Anzaldúa 1999). I began naming the *verguenza* and *culpa* I felt when I would navigate between Pocho Spanish, Spanglish, Spanish, English, and any other variation of these in my personal life and in the therapy room.

Acknowledging the emotional effects of internalizing the anti-immigrant beliefs I was exposed to since my arrival to this country allowed me to begin the journey of unlearning the shame and guilt that had been influencing my life and isolating me. I began to switch languages freely in my own life and in my clinical practice when my heart felt it necessary because picking one became too limiting. I stopped apologizing for my language. It was no longer about right or wrong; rather I finally understood that my language was the connection to *mi corazón*.

As I continued my work with the Latinx community, I witnessed the looks of relief sweep over the clients' faces when they realized I spoke Spanish and as I encouraged them to communicate in whatever language felt more comfortable for them. I made it a point to invite Spanish-/Spanglish-/Pocho Spanish-/English-speaking clients at the beginning of each session to express themselves in whatever language and variation of it their *corazón* needed. When clients would begin apologizing for their English mispronunciation and language switching, I reminded them an apology was not necessary. Suddenly, I was witnessing clients navigate their way through languages and naming the anti-immigrant systems that surrounded them. Our therapy sessions became an act of resistance, and the work we were doing was more than just about the people in the room; it was about creating change in our *comunidad*. It was small victories like these that made me realize the work I needed to do as a bilingual marriage and family therapist was more than just theories and anything graduate school had taught me; it was about using the languages I had once been made to feel ashamed of to demand change and equity.

When I sit down with a Latinx Spanish-speaking client, there is often an unspoken mutual understanding of structural inequalities, the loss accompanied with immigration, a shared culture, and a common knowledge that *no somos de aquí*. *Mi corazón bilingue* has given me the privilege to hear beautiful stories of resilience and strength, and it has also opened my eyes to how much more work still needs to be done for the Latinx community. Till today the Pocho Spanish, the Spanglish, the Spanish, and the English continue to be navigated in each session, and I hope it never stops. My many languages continue to allow me to connect with clients about telenovelas, music, food, pain, and even our shared immunization scars, but most importantly they allow me to advocate and build bridges for *mi comunidad.* Every day as I get to witness others navigate their own many languages and *corazón*, I am reminded of the power we hold with our voice and that change can only come about if we continue to utilize our tongues to demand it.

## Empowerment from a Linguistic Perspective

My name is Rocio and I was born in Cuernavaca, Morelos, Mexico. The original language of the Tlahuica people of Morelos was Nahuatl. Cuernavaca was originally Cuauhnahuac in the Nahuatl language. In Nahuatl, Cuauhnahuac means "surrounded or close by trees." Nahuatl is still spoken by 1.5 million Mexico residents. Mexico is a place with a continued history of language diversity, bilingualism, colonization, and its own language discrimination problems. Nahuatl lives in the shadows despite the millions who speak it.

When I was 5 years old, I migrated to Santa Ana, California, in 1980 to a predominantly working-class Mexican neighborhood in Orange County. I received my green card, *la mica verde*, in 1990. I returned to Cuernavaca to visit my great grandmother, Pachita, and we walked in her *Milpa* (her corn field) one last time. My heart sings when I remember her calling me *mocosa, escuincla, and chamaca.* At school predominantly white teachers punished me for speaking Spanish. Spanish at school went into hiding. I have never written these words on an academic paper before. I set them free now: *me quito los candados.*

As a result of my immigration and growing up in California, my "bilingualism" is diverse. I speak English (academic), English (slang English), Pocho Spanish, Spanglish, Standard Spanish, and working-class Mexican Spanish. My working-class clients are glad when I use certain worlds such as *trocka* (truck versus camioneta), *lonche* (lunch or almuerzo), *raite* (meaning ride versus aventon which is more street slang), and *los files* (the fields that migrant workers harvest). My upper- and middle-class Spanish speakers often remark how "well" I speak Spanish; a product of my university *Spanish* education. I witnessed language discrimination when clinicians correct clients on the "correct" usage of words (English, Spanish, or Spanglish), when intake begins in one monolingual language (Spanish or English), and when no training is given to bilingual clinicians to discuss these complexities. It is a political act for clinicians to be aware that language travels with people and that it transforms in a new land.

## Closing

In sharing our journeys and our experiences during our marriage and family therapy training and practice, we have come to understand that the MFT field needs to expand and grow to include a range of conversations about bilingualism and language discrimination. We would have welcomed more support as we negotiated language in our marriage and family therapy training. The MFT field needs to have these difficult conversations acknowledging that language diversity also has its roots in the history of colonization and racist practices, and it can also be seen in the history of the marriage and therapy field. When bilingual individuals engage in the switching of languages they are in the process of weaving their identities and they are speaking from their *corazón*. Through the use of language they are are exploring their identies, adapting, inventing and reinventing their identities and we must honor that. The training institutions owe our communities the integration of these conversations in the professional training of the new generations of MFTs. Language inclusion is an ongoing journey that all clinicians should be reflecting on and working toward.

## References

Aguilar-Gaxiola, S., Loera, G., Méndez, I., Sala, M., Latino Mental Health Concilio, & Nakamoto, J. (2012). *Community-defined solutions for Latino mental health car disparities: California reducing disparities project, Latino strategic planning workgroup population report.* Sacramento: UC Davis.

Anzaldúa, G. (1999). *Borderlands/La frontera.* San Francisco: Aunt Lute Books.

Santiago-Rivera, A. L., & Altarriba, J. (2002). The role of language in therapy with the Spanish-English bilingual client. *Professional Psychology: Research and Practice, 33*(1), 30–38. https://doi.org/10.1037/0735-7028.33.1.30.

White, M. (2006). Working with people who are suffering the consequences of multiple trauma: A narrative perspective. In D. Denborough (Ed.), *Trauma: Narrative responses to traumatic experience* (pp. 25–85). Adelaide: Dulwich Centre Publications.

# Chapter 12
# Working as a Team: Therapy with Interpreters

**Meg Rogers, Mohammed Darbi, and Jenny Leverman**

**Abstract** Though many monolingual therapists might balk at the idea of working in a second language, feeling perhaps inept or nervous at relying on a person "outside" of the therapeutic relationship for communication, we seek to provide information and examples that will help monolingual practitioners expand conceptualization of therapy to make space for interpreters in sessions. Specific logistics, including scheduling, joining, pacing, and tricky situations, will be discussed. Emphasis is placed on understanding the interpreter as a member of the therapeutic relationship, opportunities provided by deconstruction of language and assumptions of meaning uniquely facilitated by working between languages, and the importance of cultural humility in locating therapeutic practices. Examples from group, individual, and family sessions will be provided, along with reflections from the monolingual therapist authors and an interpreter. A list of logistics and learnings to consider will be provided at the end of the chapter.

We had just finished facilitating our weekly Arabic speaking men's therapy group for the Domestic Violence Intervention Program (DVIP) located at License to Freedom in El Cajon, California. I (Jenny) joined our interpreter, Mohammed, to say goodbye to our newest member. Mohammed was speaking in Arabic, repeatedly using the word *habibi* while shaking hands with him. I had heard the word before and it seemed like a term of endearment, so I shook hands with our group member and said *habibi* as well. After the whole group had dispersed, Mohammed looked at me, face solemn, and said, "You know what you just called that group member? Your lover." My breath stopped. "Mohammed, you're messing with me. Right?" He started laughing and explained that yes, the word *habibi* is a term of endearment. But it is also said between lovers in its most literal translation. This kind of cultural and linguistic meaning making is complex and can be the source of both anguish and hilarity.

M. Rogers (✉) · M. Darbi · J. Leverman
License to Freedom, El Cajon, CA, USA



m. polanco et al. (eds.), *Bilingualism, Culture, and Social Justice in Family Therapy*, AFTA SpringerBriefs in Family Therapy,
https://doi.org/10.1007/978-3-030-66036-9_12

Stories like this are common at License to Freedom, a San Diego area, community-based nonprofit which provides therapeutic services, legal advocacy, and practical support[1] at no cost for refugee/immigrant families experiencing the effects of domestic violence (DV). Most of our clients relocated to the United States from the Middle East, which means our therapy involves the work of interpreters speaking Arabic, Chaldean, and Farsi with US English. As marriage and family therapists (MFTs) increasingly engage in therapy between cultures, it is our responsibility to ensure that clients are respected, understood, and supported in the ways they prefer. As MFTs, we also have the opportunity to think systemically and create a new system within treatment. This new system could be the client-interpreter-therapist system, which could provide a model of joining cultures through communication rather than crowding out significant understandings and experiences with an expectation that a client must funnel their vast experience into English. This system could become a model to apply in social contexts outside of the therapy room. Our purpose in sharing our experiences as English-speaking therapists (Meg and Jenny) and an Arabic-speaking interpreter (Mohammed) working in collaboration with Arabic-, Chaldean-, or Farsi-speaking clients and interpreters is that readers will come away with ideas on ways to conduct therapy sessions with an interpreter, gain some practical knowledge, and have a better understanding of the complexities and benefits of working between languages. As the above story from our men's therapy group demonstrates, there is plenty of room for good humor as well. The following is a content map for this chapter: the authors' social locations, reflections from Mohammed generated by an interview about the interpreter experience conducted by Meg and Jenny, helpful practices, key ideas to working with interpreters, and additional considerations for working with couples, families, and groups.

## The Authors' Social Locations

As authors, we believe it is important to identify our social locations so that the reader might understand a little more about which languages, ideas, and discourses might be influencing our work and the ways we make meaning through therapy and interpretation. As therapists and interpreters, this acknowledgement of social locations is particularly relevant in working in the context of the United States and, more specifically, in court and DV situations, where perceived whiteness and fluency in the English language equates to power in the therapy room, in court situations, with police, and in provider interactions. As we aim to center our clients' perceptions and therapeutic experiences, we are mindful of this impact. I (Meg) am a White, middle-class, English-speaking woman and a therapist practicing from a poststructuralist (White 2007) framework. I (Mohammed) am an African/Middle Eastern, Muslim,

[1] Our clients often have to seek safety at a moment's notice; practical support includes food, clothing, transportation, and hotel vouchers.

college-educated, middle-class, Arabic–/English-speaking, single man who was raised in a family of seven siblings and both parents, valuing family, friendships, and community. I (Jenny) am a White, middle-class, English-speaking woman; my family's cultural roots are Mennonite, which inform my therapeutic practices involving community and connectedness.

## The Interpreter Experience

Interpreters at License to Freedom (LTF) are hired through a local community college's social work program, volunteer applications through CalWORKS (California's cash aid program), and through community connections to LTF's staff. Interpreters are fluent speakers of both the language they will interpret and English. When they agree to serve as interpreters, they participate in a training and sign a confidentiality agreement. Confidentiality is explained as protecting people's privacy; therapists and interpreters never share any information that could identify others. We do, however, consider ourselves the "carriers of stories" (N. Zamani, personal communication, January 16, 2020) as we engage in reflections on what is learned in people's stories and then weave this knowledge into our own lives and communities.[2] Therapists also take time to discuss with a new interpreter the purpose and focus of the therapeutic work and any intentions the therapist might hope to relay to the client.[3] We are as transparent as possible about the therapeutic process with the client and the interpreter, in order to mitigate assumed power dynamics in the therapy room. One of LTF's long-standing interpreters, who has helped shape this role at LTF, is Mohammed Darbi.

**An Interpreter's Reflection** Mohammed is a talented interpreter for the Arabic-speaking DVIP men's group and has worked at License to Freedom for nearly 4 years. In the interview with Meg and Jenny to learn more about Mohammed's experience for the purpose of this chapter, he reflected that building trust with the men is a key aspect in the interpreter-client relationship and that joining group members on their 10-minute break has been a connective practice. During those breaks, there is space for personal conversations. "We teach each other. I learn a lot from them." Mohammed shared what has been meaningful in his work as an interpreter. "I get to really understand what they say – what they say and what they mean." An example was translating the English phrase "walking on eggshells" to the Arabic phrase "walking on tiptoes." He bridges these cultural understandings and emphasizes that, "In my mind, I carry not just words but the emotions."

[2] We have seen the client-interpreter-therapist system create awareness and activism around DV and connect people in unexpected, beautiful ways as the stories throughout this chapter will attest.

[3] An example might be "I'm going to ask questions, and not make statements, so feel free to express my ideas as questions throughout our meeting."

To best facilitate conversation, Mohammed asks everyone to take breaks as they are speaking so that he "can get every detail of a touching story." He added, "Summarizing is less effective." He also noted the importance of being tolerant. "You'll hear a lot of offensive things, things that don't make sense, and things you don't agree with." He has witnessed the effects of this group on his personal life and spoke about his awareness around DV and spreading this awareness. "I passed what I learned [in group] to my friends and they took it positively." Mohammed shared that sometimes his mind would drift into memories during the group because he was thinking about his own family. "This group made me realize that my mom was in a DV [relationship] for 33 years." This awareness has shifted to activism: he believes that what is learned in the community of the group should then be spread to the community at large. "I'm proud of what I'm doing there. It's changed me, and changed my mom's life in a totally different direction. I thank the group for that."

## Helpful Practices

Throughout our work with interpreters, we three (Mohammed, Jenny, and Meg) have come to identify a few specific helpful practices that contribute to our therapy work across languages with families who speak Arabic, Chaldean, or Farsi.

- In the small Arabic-speaking community of San Diego, we offer demographic descriptions of interpreters to the client so that they can avoid any relatives, friends, or other community connections as interpreters. No third cousins four times removed!
- When scheduling a client, we always ask for their language preference. We leave this decision up to clients: some wish to work in English and some in Arabic, Chaldean, or Farsi.[4] If an interpreter will be joining the session, we clarify any regional preferences.[5]
- We hold a mindset of "I wish I spoke Arabic," instead of "I wish you spoke English." Our clients speak multiple languages and we speak one.
- We make copies of our client's ID or court documents when necessary. This saves time as the interpreter does not need to interpret, for instance, every number on a driver's license.
- For the initial contact, we call clients to set up appointments with an interpreter on the phone. This can be managed by merging phone lines.

[4] I (Meg) find this relates as much to how the client wishes to understand themselves and their experience, as much as fluency in any language. I have heard "It is easier to think about this in English" and "It happened in Arabic, so that makes sense for me."

[5] For example, people speak English in Scotland differently than people speak English in the United States or New Zealand. This is represented in accent, colloquialisms, and even specific words that do not exist outside of a specific region but are still English. The same concept applies to the languages our clients speak.

- During our first session, the interpreter signs a confidentiality form and we explain what confidentiality in a therapy context is, in depth to our client. This goes a long way in putting clients at ease.
- At the end of each session, we schedule our next session while the interpreter is present.
- Caring for our interpreters is of great importance to us. We create space after therapy sessions for interpreters to share any personal reflections.
- We have seen that in the midst of varying linguistic/cultural contexts with our clients and interpreters, agility and good humor create the conditions necessary for connection.

## Key Ideas to Working with Interpreters

**Pacing** In conducting therapy with interpreters, we have experienced the slowness of the sessions as rich in possibilities. While translations are being made, there is time to think about a question one might pose or time to really notice the nonverbal actions of the client and their affect. There is breathing room. Sessions often go longer because of the time it takes to communicate effectively, so we allow for this in our scheduling. An hour session often requires 2 hours.[6]

**Interpreter as a Witness to Stories** Each member of the therapy system is involved in both building meaning through words and adding meaning through listening. This meaning becomes more profound when an interpreter witnesses the story as a person of a similar cultural background, understanding the depths of the client's contexts that could not be assumed by the different-cultured therapist.

I (Jenny) was in session with a client and interpreter discussing the client's service in the Iraqi army when he was a young man. His stories were particularly moving for us all; the client hadn't spoken of these memories in decades. The interpreter arrived early the next week to share with me that this session had prompted her to call her father in Iraq, who was the same age as this client. She had asked her father, "Did you participate in this war? Did all that happen to *you*? Were *you* hungry, afraid, hopeless?" Her father answered yes to her questions and shared his experiences. She then asked him why he had never told her before. He said, "I did not want you to be sad." She shared how touched she had been by this conversation with her father and I asked if she would like to share this with our client. She agreed and in session that day told our client about this connective conversation. Our client smiled, emotion in his eyes, because he understood her father's intentions. There was a common experience and cultural value that was being upheld: seeking happiness for one's children. This is but one of many moments when interpreters' experiences and

---

[6] Depending on a therapist's means of collecting payment and schedule management, this may be an issue to address with insurance and clients at the outset of treatment.

meaning making render a "portrait of culture *happening*" (m. polanco, personal communication, February 20, 2020).

**Negotiating Meaning Through Interpretation Across Languages** Although interpreters share points of linguistic, and often cultural, similarity with clients, there is also room for differences of opinions and understandings of words, which can be rich territory for therapeutic discovery. In one opportunity, an Iraqi, Arabic-speaking woman presented for therapy to organize her thoughts around experiences of DV and to determine how she could move forward with family relationships in a way that made sense for her values. We (Meg, the client, and the interpreter) came to an understanding that jealousy was playing a large role in her relationships with other women, who might otherwise be a support to her and was making her feel inferior. At the start of our relationship, we began laying out elements of the client's story on a metaphorical table: like many puzzle pieces that connected in the client's mind and experience, but we, as a group, were unsure how they connected or what meaning might be developed from their connection. By taking time with each piece, comparing them, finding patterns, and drawing connections, we located a central theme of "jealousy." Jealousy was directly impacting her relationship with her Iraqi husband and influencing the way in-laws positioned her in relationship to other woman family members, but each story and puzzle piece representing "jealousy" looked different.

My (Meg) English-speaking brain would have labeled these pieces with words other than jealousy and would have lost connections between the stories. With our interpreter, the client and I spent time considering definitions of words, describing physical sensations we connected with meanings, and finding similar experiences to help illustrate points. We knew when we hit on a moment of resonance and understanding when our interpreter would sit up a little straighter, smile, and make a comment such as "Oh, ok, now we have it!" As a richness of lived experiences developed, and through our interpreter's skill, we were able to come to the consensus that these seemingly disparate pieces were all influenced by jealousy. I did not realize the depth of meaning jealousy held, or the nuances of jealousy, in Iraqi culture, but the interpreter did. We did not have to settle for misunderstanding, or half understandings, as our trusted interpreter was able to let us know when we hit on something important, in both English and Arabic, dramatically improving the quality of experience for all involved.

## Additional Considerations for Family and Couples Therapy

Family and couples therapy can be supported by skilled interpreters and also has the potential to run wildly amok. Interpreters can slow the process of therapy and explanations down, which can benefit the therapeutic process by allowing clients who are heightened to self-regulate and consider exactly which words they would like to use to convey meaning.

This is not to say that conflict cannot occur within sessions and cannot be managed with the support of interpreters. A common theme in couples presenting for therapy is that one partner has more facility with English than the other partner. The client not speaking English can feel left out that we are "talking about" them and overwhelmed. Frequent reminders to pause and turn to the interpreter are required, and I (Meg) am clear with the interpreter before the session that everything, no matter how seemingly inconsequential, spoken in English must be interpreted. Noticing the leverage of linguistic power and communication patterns can be extremely useful in identifying habits of communication, particularly in a DV context. This can also be a powerful influence when considering sessions between English-speaking children and native language-speaking parents. We are mindful of the power dynamics in family therapy when children speak English and parents speak Arabic: we ensure that everything is translated by the interpreter in order for everyone to understand. We avoid having children interpret for their parents.

Pauses to interpret and reminders to involve the language other than English can be playfully or kindly positioned. I've heard interpreters make comments like "I'm so sorry, there's so much, I want to get it just right." This relational approach to navigating the power of language builds trust, a therapeutic alliance, and has the potential to shift power dynamics within a relationship. When I (Meg) am called on to shift focus and allow the interpreter space to do their work, I employ similar language: "Wait, wait! I need to catch up, this is all so important, can you please help me understand?"

## Additional Considerations for Groups

Our men's DVIP group includes approximately eight court-mandated clients, three therapists, and one interpreter. Most clients speak a number of languages, including English, but all in varying degrees. We have found it helpful to limit the conversation to two languages: in our case, Arabic and English. Mohammed requested the fluent Arabic speakers to speak Arabic to him and he would translate to English and vice versa with the fluent English speakers. This created a much easier flow of conversation. When speaking in group, we all pause every minute or so in order for Mohammed to interpret. Each member is encouraged to respect the voices of others and wait to speak in order that their own voice be heard as well. One intention of the group is to collectively learn how to be in respectful disagreement, where we listen not just to respond but to really understand one another. The interpreter's work within the group provides an opportunity to see this community ethic in practice.

## Closing Remarks

While it may at first glance seem daunting to engage in therapy with an interpreter, we have found the experience to be illuminating and just plain fun. MFTs play an integral role in building relational bridges in our communities; the client-interpreter-therapist system can provide a model of teamwork that gives pause to assumptions and strives for deeper meaning within relationships, long after therapy is concluded.

## Reference

White, M. (2007). *Maps of narrative practice*. New York: W.W. Norton & Company.

# Index





m. polanco et al. (eds.), *Bilingualism, Culture, and Social Justice in Family Therapy*, AFTA SpringerBriefs in Family Therapy,
https://doi.org/10.1007/978-3-030-66036-9

**W**

The manufacturer's authorised representative in the EU is Springer Nature Customer Service Centre GmbH, Europaplatz 3, 69115 Heidelberg, Germany. If you have any concerns regarding our products, please contact ProductSafety@springernature.com

Printed and bound by CPI Group (UK) Ltd, Croydon, CR0 4YY
28/09/2026
02224076-0013